Digestive Emergencies

A Practical Guide for Rapid Diagnosis and Treatment

Dr. Ewan Gregory

Chapter 1
Introduction to Digestive Emergencies

Understanding the Landscape of Digestive Emergencies

Digestive emergencies represent a complex and critical domain within acute care medicine, encompassing a wide array of conditions that require immediate attention and intervention. From subtle presentations like dysphagia to dramatic, life-threatening events such as acute liver failure or severe gastrointestinal bleeding, the spectrum of digestive emergencies is both diverse and challenging. These conditions demand not only clinical expertise but also a structured and evidence-based approach to ensure accurate diagnosis, timely treatment, and optimal patient outcomes.

This book, Digestive Emergencies: A Practical Guide for Rapid Diagnosis and Treatment, is meticulously designed to serve as a comprehensive reference and practical guide for healthcare providers managing these high-stakes scenarios.

Purpose and Objectives

The purpose of this book is to provide healthcare professionals—ranging from emergency physicians to specialists in gastroenterology and surgery—with a focused resource for addressing digestive emergencies. Its objectives include:

1. Systematic Approach: Offering clear, step-by-step methodologies for evaluating and managing common and uncommon digestive conditions.

2. Rapid Decision-Making: Equipping clinicians with tools like flowcharts, diagnostic algorithms, and checklists to enhance efficiency.

3. Evidence-Based Care: Integrating the latest clinical guidelines, research, and best practices into the diagnostic and therapeutic framework.

Book Structure and Highlights

This book is organized into 15 chapters, each dedicated to a specific topic within the realm of digestive emergencies. The chapters follow a logical progression, beginning with fundamental approaches and moving into specific conditions.

- Chapter 1: Introduction
Sets the stage with an overview of the importance of digestive emergency management, the challenges faced by clinicians, and the interdisciplinary nature of care.

- Chapter 2: Dysphagia
Covers the diagnostic approach to difficulty swallowing, including key red flags for esophageal obstruction, motility disorders, and structural anomalies.

- Chapter 3: Approach to Abdominal Pain
Introduces a systematic evaluation of abdominal pain, emphasizing differential diagnosis, physical examination, and key investigations.

- Chapter 4: Bowel Obstruction
Discusses the types, causes, and management strategies for mechanical and functional obstructions of the bowel.

- Chapter 5: Herniae
Explores the identification and management of hernias, focusing on complications such as strangulation and incarceration.

- Chapter 6: Gastroenteritis
Examines infectious and non-infectious causes of gastroenteritis, with a focus on rehydration and targeted treatment.

- Chapter 7: Haematemesis and Melaena

Details the evaluation and management of upper gastrointestinal bleeding, including endoscopic interventions and stabilization protocols.

- Chapter 8: Peptic Ulcer Disease Management
Reviews the pathophysiology, diagnosis, and treatment of peptic ulcers and their complications.

- Chapter 9: Biliary Tract Disease
Addresses conditions like cholecystitis, cholangitis, and biliary obstruction, with a focus on diagnostic imaging and surgical options.

- Chapter 10: Acute Pancreatitis
Highlights the management of mild to severe acute pancreatitis, including fluid resuscitation, pain control, and treatment of complications.

- Chapter 11: Acute Appendicitis
Describes the clinical presentation, diagnostic tools, and surgical management of one of the most common abdominal emergencies.

- Chapter 12: Inflammatory Bowel Disease
Discusses the acute exacerbations of Crohn's disease and ulcerative colitis, focusing on medical and surgical management.

- Chapter 13: Acute Liver Failure (ALF)
Examines the critical care of patients with ALF, including identification of causes, supportive therapies, and indications for transplantation.

- Chapter 14: Hematochezia and Lower Gastrointestinal Bleeding (LGIB)
Explores the approach to bright red bleeding per rectum, emphasizing stabilization, diagnosis, and endoscopic interventions.

- Chapter 15: Perianal Conditions Management
Provides guidance on the evaluation and treatment of perianal abscesses, fissures, fistulas, and other common conditions.

Key Features of the Book

Practical Algorithms: Step-by-step diagnostic and treatment protocols tailored for emergency settings.

Visual Aids: Flowcharts, tables, and high-yield illustrations to simplify complex processes.

Clinical Insights: Pearls and pitfalls based on real-world cases and expert experience.

Case-Based Learning: Scenarios that contextualize theoretical knowledge into practical applications.

Intended Audience

This book is an essential resource for:

Emergency Physicians and Residents: To manage acute digestive emergencies with confidence and precision.

Gastroenterologists and Surgeons: To refine their diagnostic and therapeutic skills in critical situations.

Medical Students and Trainees: To build foundational knowledge and gain exposure to practical aspects of digestive emergency care.

Conclusion

Digestive Emergencies: A Practical Guide for Rapid Diagnosis and Treatment is more than just a reference—it is a hands-on manual for navigating the complexities of digestive emergencies. With its systematic structure, evidence-based content, and practical focus, this book is designed to empower clinicians at all levels to deliver timely, effective, and life-saving care. Dr. Ewan Gregory's expertise ensures that this guide is not only comprehensive but also accessible and impactful, setting a new standard for resources in digestive emergency management.

Chapter 2
Dysphagia

1. Dysphagia presents a diagnostic challenge and requires a broad differential diagnosis. A thorough patient history often provides critical clues to identify the underlying cause.

2. Dysphagia resulting from acute conditions like a recent stroke, or pharyngeal or esophageal disorders, can lead to food accumulation in the pharynx, increasing the risk of aspiration. Assessing this risk is essential before allowing oral intake.

3. Patients experiencing chronic or prolonged dysphagia may develop significant fluid and electrolyte imbalances along with severe nutritional deficiencies.

4. Emergency department evaluations should focus on identifying high-grade obstructions or lesions that pose immediate threats, such as airway compromise, hemorrhage, or sepsis.

5. Psychological causes of dysphagia are exceedingly rare, with almost all cases attributable to physical conditions.

Introduction to Dysphagia

Dysphagia refers to a range of difficulties in swallowing. Effective management involves identifying the underlying cause, assessing the risk of complications, initiating appropriate treatments for conditions that can be addressed acutely, and ensuring timely referrals for further evaluation and management. Dysphagia is often accompanied by odynophagia (painful swallowing), while globus refers to the sensation of a lump in the throat, which is seldom psychological in origin. Modern diagnostic methods have revealed that most cases have an identifiable physical cause.

Etiology

Dysphagia arises from problems in one or more stages of swallowing: oral, pharyngeal, or esophageal.

Oral/Pharyngeal Dysphagia: Often categorized as transfer dysphagia, caused by issues like muscle coordination deficits or neurological disorders.

Esophageal Dysphagia: Known as transport dysphagia, typically due to structural obstructions (e.g., tumors) or motility disorders.

Medications can also contribute to dysphagia. Common offenders include tetracyclines, NSAIDs, ascorbic acid, potassium chloride, and iron supplements. A detailed drug history is crucial in evaluating these cases.

Clinical Presentation

Symptoms may develop gradually or manifest acutely.

Acute Presentation: Obstruction from impacted food boluses may result in severe retching, drooling, pain, or the inability to swallow saliva.

Chronic Symptoms: Gradual progression from difficulty swallowing solids to liquids is typical, though some cases may lack prior dysphagia history.

Key indicators include coughing or hoarseness after meals, which are sensitive signs of aspiration. Patients with recent cerebrovascular events should be presumed dysphagic until swallowing is formally assessed. Pulse oximetry desaturation, however, is not a reliable indicator of aspiration.

Examination should evaluate cranial nerve function, hydration, nutritional status, and signs of sepsis or perforation. A history of ingesting sharp objects or corrosive substances warrants additional attention, with surgical emphysema in the neck indicating possible perforation.

Clinical Investigations

Diagnostic approaches depend on the clinical context:

Radiology: Plain chest or neck X-rays are helpful for radiopaque foreign bodies, while CT is preferred for non-opaque materials or suspected perforation.

Specialized Tests: Endoscopy and video fluoroscopy are key for semi-elective cases, but barium studies should be avoided if endoscopy is planned.

Laboratory Studies: Basic biochemistry and blood work help detect dehydration, electrolyte imbalances, or anemia.

Management

Treatment strategies depend on the underlying cause and severity of symptoms:

Emergency Interventions: Patients with high-grade obstructions require immediate cessation of oral intake and IV fluid administration if symptoms persist. Endoscopic removal of sharp objects or bolus impactions is recommended within 2–6 hours for severe cases, or within 24 hours for minor cases. Medical interventions with glucagon or GTN may help but often have limited efficacy.

Foreign Body Removal: Pharyngeal obstructions (e.g., bones) may be addressed in the ED using topical anesthetics and direct laryngoscopy.

Complications: Esophageal or pharyngeal perforations necessitate broad-spectrum antibiotics and urgent surgical consultation.

Pain management includes topical or parenteral analgesia, such as viscous lidocaine, with dose adjustments for elderly patients to minimize systemic risks.

Disposition

Admission is required for patients with risks such as airway compromise, significant hemorrhage, sepsis, or high-grade obstruction. Outpatient referrals to gastroenterologists should be arranged for patients with resolved symptoms for further evaluation, including elective endoscopy.

Controversies and Emerging Evidence

1. Diet Modifications: Recent studies suggest that altering food consistency in patients with chronic dysphagia, particularly the elderly, does not reduce pulmonary complications.

2. Long-Term Aspiration Management: The severity of aspiration does not consistently correlate with survival outcomes, raising questions about the benefits of prolonged interventions.

References

1. Balzer, K. M. (2000). Drug-induced dysphagia. International Journal of MS Care, 2(1), 40–50.

2. Sassi, F. C., Medeiros, G. C., Zilberstein, B., et al. (2017). Screening protocol for dysphagia in adults: Comparison with videofluoroscopic findings. Clinics (São Paulo), 72(12), 718–722.

3. Britton, D., Roeske, A., Ennis, S. K., et al. (2018). Utility of pulse oximetry to detect

aspiration: An evidence-based systematic review. Dysphagia, 33(3), 282–292.

4. Johnston, B. T. (2017). Esophageal dysphagia: A stepwise approach to diagnosis and management. The Lancet Gastroenterology & Hepatology, 2(8), 604–609.

5. Birk, M., Bauerfield, P., Deprez, P. H., et al. (2016). Removal of foreign bodies in the upper gastrointestinal tract in adults: European Society of Gastrointestinal Endoscopy (ESGE) Clinical Guideline. Endoscopy, 48(5), 489–496.

6. Sodeman, T. C., Harewood, G. C., & Baron, T. H. (2004). Assessment of predictors of response to glucagon in acute esophageal food bolus obstruction. Dysphagia, 19, 18–21.

7. Bock, J. A., Varadarajan, V., Brawly, M. C., & Blumin, J. H. (2017). Evaluation of the natural history of patients who aspirate. Laryngoscope, 127(Suppl 8), S1–S10.

Chapter 3
Approach to Abdominal Pain

Essentials

1. Abdominal pain is responsible for approximately 4% to 10% of all visits to the emergency department.

2. While gastrointestinal and genitourinary pathologies are the most common sources of abdominal pain, it can also stem from cardiovascular, respiratory, metabolic, infectious, or toxic conditions.

3. Special populations, including the elderly, immunocompromised individuals, obese patients, women of reproductive age, and children, require meticulous evaluation to prevent misdiagnosis and adverse outcomes.

4. In 25% to 40% of cases, the precise cause of abdominal pain may remain undetermined in the emergency setting. Decisions regarding admission, discharge, or extended observation should be guided by symptom management, potential diagnoses, and the patient's risk factors.

5. Patients presenting with abdominal pain should receive appropriate analgesia, including opioids when necessary. Proper pain management facilitates accurate diagnosis and does not obscure signs indicative of an acute abdomen.

Comprehensive Analysis and Approach to Abdominal Pain Management in Emergency Settings

Introduction

Abdominal pain is a frequent and complex presentation in emergency departments (EDs), often stemming from a diverse range of potential causes. Effective assessment aims to identify the underlying cause while prioritizing the exclusion of acute, life-threatening conditions and ensuring appropriate patient disposition. Definitive diagnosis may not always be achievable during initial evaluation, necessitating decisions based on clinical risk assessment, patient characteristics, and the likelihood of specific conditions.

The evaluation of abdominal pain is particularly challenging due to several factors:

Early-stage symptoms and signs are often nonspecific.

Presentation can vary widely, especially in pediatric, elderly, immunocompromised, or obese patients.

Pain severity and physical findings may not correlate with the underlying pathology.

Epidemiology, Pathophysiology, and Differential Diagnosis

Abdominal pain accounts for 4% to 10% of ED visits, with 18% to 42% of these patients requiring hospital admission. Among older individuals, the need for surgical intervention (18% to 20%) and mortality risk are significantly higher.

Patterns of Abdominal Pain:

1. Visceral Pain:

Originates from nociceptor activation in internal organs (e.g., gut, biliary system, pancreas).

Typically diffuse and poorly localized, correlating to embryological organ segments (e.g., foregut pain in the upper abdomen, midgut in the periumbilical region).

Causes include obstruction, ischemia, and inflammation.

2. Parietal Pain:

Stems from stimulation of nociceptors in the parietal peritoneum or abdominal wall structures.

Pain is sharp, well-localized, and often indicative of intra-abdominal inflammation, such as appendicitis or generalized peritonitis.

3. Referred Pain:

Occurs at a distant site due to shared spinal innervation. Examples include:

Shoulder pain from diaphragmatic irritation.

Scapular pain due to gallbladder pathology.

Epigastric discomfort associated with myocardial infarction.

Generalized Abdominal Pain:
Encompasses a broad differential, ranging from benign conditions to critical emergencies. Non-abdominal causes, such as diabetic ketoacidosis, vasculitis, or pulmonary embolism, must also be considered.

Clinical Features of Abdominal Pain

Patient History:
A focused history provides vital diagnostic clues. Key aspects include:

Risk Factors: Prior surgeries, body habitus, or conditions affecting assessment, such as renal impairment.

Demographics: Age and gender predispose patients to specific conditions (e.g., biliary disease in women aged 35–50; mesenteric ischemia in the elderly).

Symptoms: Onset, progression, location, severity, and nature of pain offer insights into potential etiologies. For example, pain migrating from the umbilicus to the right iliac fossa suggests appendicitis.

Associated Symptoms: Nausea, vomiting, or changes in bowel or urinary habits may refine the differential diagnosis.

Pain Characteristics:

Onset and Progression: Acute vascular events, like aortic aneurysm rupture, typically present with sudden, severe pain, whereas inflammatory conditions evolve gradually.

Severity: Pain perception varies; elderly patients often exhibit attenuated pain responses, necessitating early intervention despite mild symptoms.

Precipitating Factors: Pain exacerbated by movement may indicate peritonitis, while postprandial discomfort suggests biliary colic or peptic ulcer disease.

Physical Examination

A structured examination corroborates historical findings and may reveal unexpected abnormalities:

1. General Appearance: Signs such as pallor, jaundice, or dehydration provide systemic clues. Patient posture may indicate underlying conditions (e.g., stillness in peritonitis vs. restlessness in renal colic).

2. Abdominal Inspection: Note distension, visible peristalsis, or surgical scars.

3. Palpation: Localized tenderness (e.g., Murphy's sign for cholecystitis), rebound tenderness, or guarding suggests peritoneal irritation.

4. Special Tests: Consider rectal, pelvic, or scrotal examinations when clinically indicated to localize pathology.

Clinical Investigations: A Comprehensive Analysis

Clinical investigations are vital for diagnosing, monitoring, and evaluating patient responses to treatment. They assist in identifying or excluding pathologies, gauging a patient's condition, and screening for coexisting conditions. Effective investigations should address specific clinical questions, with results interpreted within the broader clinical and diagnostic context. Importantly, negative findings do not always exclude serious conditions in patients with high pre-test probabilities.

Bedside Testing

Blood Gas Analysis

Blood gas analysis rapidly evaluates acid-base balance and other critical parameters like hemoglobin, electrolytes, creatinine, glucose, and lactate. Elevated lactate levels often indicate tissue hypoxia, whether from systemic hypoperfusion or localized ischemia. However, normal lactate levels cannot exclude conditions like ischemic bowel, as sensitivities for intestinal ischemia remain as low as 70%.

Urine Analysis

Urine analysis offers early diagnostic clues for urinary tract infections (UTIs) and ureteric colic. However, results must align with clinical findings, as conditions like acute appendicitis (30% prevalence of blood or leukocytes in urine) or ruptured abdominal aortic aneurysms (30% incidence of hematuria) can present atypically.

Conversely, up to one-third of patients with urolithiasis may lack hematuria.

Pregnancy Testing

Rapid and highly sensitive bedside urine pregnancy tests detect β-human chorionic gonadotropin (β-hCG) levels as low as 25 mU/mL. However, up to 1% of ectopic pregnancies involve β-hCG values below this threshold, requiring clinical correlation.

Electrocardiography (ECG)

ECG is essential for older patients with abdominal pain, as cardiac ischemia or arrhythmias can manifest as abdominal symptoms like epigastric pain, nausea, or vomiting. Furthermore, ECG findings may point to causes like mesenteric ischemia in atrial fibrillation or digoxin toxicity presenting with abdominal symptoms.

Laboratory Tests

Full Blood Count (FBC)

FBC is a standard test but has limitations. A normal white blood cell count does not rule out conditions like appendicitis, seen in 10–60% of cases, or severe intra-abdominal pathology, where only 50% of patients exhibit leukocytosis. Conversely, an elevated count is nonspecific and may indicate various inflammatory conditions.

Electrolytes

Electrolyte assessment rarely provides a direct diagnosis, although hypercalcemia can present with abdominal pain.

Liver Function Tests (LFTs)

LFT abnormalities are observed in hepatobiliary disorders, sepsis, or other systemic conditions and may influence treatment strategies.

Lipase

An elevated lipase level three times above normal is diagnostic of acute pancreatitis. However, elevated lipase levels can also result from other pathologies like renal dysfunction or salivary gland disorders. Conversely, lipase levels may remain normal in CT-confirmed cases of recurrent pancreatitis.

C-Reactive Protein (CRP)

As an acute-phase reactant, CRP is elevated in inflammation and can aid in monitoring conditions like appendicitis. However, its utility varies, emphasizing the need for serial measurements in some cases.

Imaging Modalities

Plain X-Rays

While their diagnostic value is limited, plain radiographs (erect chest, supine abdomen) are useful in suspected bowel obstruction, perforation, or foreign body cases. Findings are specific but lack sensitivity, helping confirm but not exclude diagnoses.

Ultrasound (US)

Ultrasound is a first-line diagnostic tool with extensive applications in emergency settings. It is operator-dependent and requires appropriate training for accurate results.

Hemoperitoneum: The FAST (Focused Abdominal Sonography in Trauma) protocol is critical for unstable trauma patients, offering 99% specificity for hemoperitoneum but with variable sensitivity (66%).

Abdominal Aortic Aneurysm (AAA): Ultrasound enables rapid AAA identification, crucial for unstable patients unsuitable for CT.

Gallbladder Disease & Pelvic Pathologies: Ultrasound remains the preferred modality for assessing gallbladder conditions, tubo-ovarian diseases, and ectopic pregnancies.

Computed Tomography (CT)

CT has become the gold standard for evaluating abdominal pain in non-obstetric patients, offering precise visualization of intra-abdominal structures. It achieves diagnostic accuracy in over 95% of cases. However, its limitations include ionizing radiation exposure, nephrotoxicity risks, and delayed intervention in surgical emergencies.

Magnetic Resonance Imaging (MRI)
MRI excels in soft tissue visualization and avoids radiation, making it ideal for hepatobiliary conditions, mesenteric ischemia, and appendicitis. However, its limited availability, cost, and contraindications restrict routine use in acute settings.

Imaging in Special Populations

Pregnancy
Ultrasound remains the safest modality during pregnancy. MRI is also considered safe, though gadolinium-based contrast agents should be avoided. While CT is reserved for specific

indications, its radiation levels are generally below harmful thresholds for fetal development.

Elderly Patients

Elderly individuals are at greater risk for surgical conditions, complications, and delayed diagnoses. Presenting atypically, they often require a lower threshold for imaging, surgical consultation, and admission to improve outcomes.

Patient Disposition and Management in the Emergency Department

Criteria for Discharge

Patients may be safely discharged from the emergency department (ED) if they meet the following criteria:

1. No Immediate Need for Inpatient Care: There is no confirmed or highly suspected diagnosis necessitating acute hospitalization.

2. Favorable Social Conditions: The patient's social circumstances are supportive of recovery and follow-up.

3. Ability to Return: The patient can seek medical attention promptly if symptoms worsen.

4. No Anticipated Deterioration: The clinical course is expected to remain stable without sudden decline.

Patients who fail to meet these criteria should remain under hospital care. This may involve admission to an inpatient unit or monitoring in an emergency observation unit, especially when a non-critical diagnosis is expected. Observation allows for:

Serial examinations to refine diagnosis.

Monitoring response to initial treatments.

Early identification of acute abdominal pathology.

Additional diagnostic evaluations as necessary.

Discharge Instructions

Discharge advice is critical, as some conditions may evolve after the initial ED visit. Patients should be instructed to return to the ED if they experience any of the following:

Persistent or worsening pain lasting beyond 24 hours.

Severe vomiting or inability to retain fluids.

Progression of vague pain to localized pain (e.g., right iliac fossa).

Development of high fever, chills, or feeling increasingly unwell.

Episodes of fainting or significant weakness.

Abdominal distension.

Presence of blood in stool or vomit.

New or worsening medical issues requiring urgent evaluation.

Non-Specific Abdominal Pain (NSAP)

A significant proportion of patients discharged with abdominal pain do not have a definitive diagnosis:

Younger Adults (<50 years): NSAP accounts for approximately 40% of cases and generally has a benign course.

Elderly Patients: NSAP is less common (about 15%) but poses a higher risk of underlying malignancy (~10% of cases).

For younger, stable patients whose symptoms resolve after treatment and observation, discharge with clear instructions is often appropriate. They should be informed that the exact cause of their symptoms was not determined and advised to return if symptoms recur or worsen. Specialist referral for further evaluation may be recommended. In elderly patients, clinicians should also consider extra-abdominal causes.

Advances in Abdominal Pain Management

Emerging Diagnostic Tools for Acute Mesenteric Ischemia (AMI)

Early detection and surgical intervention significantly enhance outcomes in AMI. However, diagnosis in early stages remains challenging.

CT imaging is the primary diagnostic tool, while lactate levels, although commonly used, are non-specific.

Novel biomarkers like citrulline have shown promise in improving diagnostic accuracy, but further research is needed to establish clinical thresholds and marker combinations for broader application.

Controversies in Abdominal Pain Management

1. Clinical Scoring Systems

Tools such as the Alvarado score for suspected appendicitis promote systematic evaluation. However, no scoring system has demonstrated superiority to physician judgment in prospective studies.

2. Antibiotic Management of Uncomplicated Appendicitis

Meta-analyses on conservative treatment with antibiotics versus surgical intervention have yielded conflicting conclusions regarding safety and efficacy, highlighting the need for individualized patient management.

Chapter 4
Bowel Obstruction

Essentials

1. Etiology

Small Bowel Obstruction (SBO): Predominantly arises due to adhesions, hernias, or tumors.

Large Bowel Obstruction (LBO): Commonly results from malignancies, volvulus, or strictures.

2. Clinical Features

Symptoms include intermittent, poorly localized abdominal pain, constipation or obstipation, abdominal distension, nausea, vomiting, and hyperactive or high-pitched bowel sounds.

A thorough examination for hernias is critical.

3. Imaging Diagnosis

Abdominal X-rays: Typically reveal dilated bowel loops with multiple air-fluid levels, confirming the obstruction.

CT Scan: Recommended if clinical suspicion is strong but plain radiographs are inconclusive.

4. Initial Management

Key steps involve correcting dehydration and electrolyte imbalances, decompressing the bowel, providing pain relief, and performing further evaluations, particularly for suspected strangulation.

5. Surgical Indications

Urgent surgery is required for cases involving strangulated bowel obstruction or bowel perforation.

Introduction and Pathophysiology of Bowel Obstruction

Bowel obstruction is a medical condition characterized by the disruption of normal intestinal content transit. It may result from either a mechanical obstruction or functional failure of intestinal motility without a clear blockage. Obstructions can affect either the small or large bowel and are classified as partial or complete, and strangulating or non-strangulating.

Causes

For small bowel obstruction (SBO), the most common causes are summarized by the mnemonic ABC:

Adhesions (60%–85%)

Bulge (hernia, 2%–3%)

Cancer/Crohn's Disease (neoplasms 2%–5%, Crohn's 5%–7%)

Other less frequent causes include gallstones, foreign bodies, strictures, radiation injury, diverticulitis, endometriosis, and abscesses. Large bowel obstruction (LBO) is primarily caused by adenocarcinoma (90%), volvulus, and strictures from diverticulitis.

Pathophysiology

Mechanical obstructions cause increased intraluminal pressure, leading to:

1. Distension of the proximal bowel with gas, fluid, and electrolytes.

2. Reduced absorptive ability and increased secretions.

3. Systemic volume depletion due to fluid losses, further aggravated by vomiting, especially in proximal obstructions.

If the obstruction persists, venous stasis and vascular compromise occur, raising the risk of ischemia, strangulation, necrosis, and eventual perforation with systemic sepsis. A closed-loop obstruction—where both proximal and distal segments are obstructed—carries a particularly high risk of ischemia and perforation due to rapid vascular compromise.

In functional obstruction, motility failure occurs without physical blockage, often due to postoperative adynamic ileus or Ogilvie syndrome (acute colonic pseudo-obstruction). Risk factors include certain medications (e.g., calcium channel blockers, anticholinergics), severe electrolyte imbalances, neurological conditions, thyroid disorders, acute illnesses, or recent surgeries.

Clinical Features of Bowel Obstruction

History

Pain Characteristics:

Initially colicky and poorly localized.

Becomes constant and severe if ischemia, strangulation, or perforation develops.

Associated Symptoms:

Proximal SBO: Frequent vomiting, minimal distension, rapid onset of symptoms.

Distal SBO/LBO: Progressive abdominal distension, delayed vomiting, and obstipation.

Feculent vomiting suggests a high-grade SBO.

Additional Clues:

Gastrointestinal and surgical history (e.g., prior surgeries suggest adhesions).

Medication history may reveal causes of functional obstruction.

Physical Examination

Key findings include:

Abdominal distension, particularly in distal SBO and LBO.

Bowel sounds: High-pitched "tinkling" sounds or absent sounds in late stages.

Palpable mass: May indicate a tumor or hernia.

Signs of vascular compromise: Fever, tachycardia, localized tenderness, or peritonitis.

Rectal and pelvic examinations are critical for detecting masses, blood, or abscesses and for evaluating gynecological causes in females.

Diagnostic Investigations

Laboratory Testing

Non-specific markers: Elevated hematocrit (dehydration) and inflammatory markers (e.g., C-reactive protein).

Electrolyte imbalances: Hyponatremia, hypokalemia, and metabolic acidosis.

Rising lactate: Indicates ischemia.

Imaging

1. Abdominal X-rays (AXRs):

Dilated bowel loops and air-fluid levels are characteristic.

Sensitivity: Variable for SBO (59%–93%); less reliable for closed-loop or strangulated obstructions.

Volvulus features: "Bent inner-tube" (sigmoid) or "kidney bean" (cecal).

2. Computed Tomography (CT):

High sensitivity and specificity for SBO (90%–95%) and LBO (96%).

Identifies ischemia via signs like intramural gas or mesenteric fluid.

3. Ultrasound: Emerging as a bedside tool with promising sensitivity.

4. MRI: Less practical in emergencies due to limited availability.

Management Strategies

General Measures

Fluid resuscitation with crystalloid solutions to address dehydration and electrolyte imbalances.

Nasogastric decompression to alleviate discomfort and prevent aspiration.

Analgesia: IV opioids are preferred.

Conservative Therapy

For stable patients with partial obstruction:

Continue IV fluids, bowel rest, and monitor clinical progress.

Use water-soluble contrast agents like Gastrografin to aid resolution in adhesive SBO.

Surgical Intervention

Surgery is warranted for:

Complete obstruction, strangulation, or perforation.

Options include laparotomy or laparoscopic adhesiolysis, depending on the pathology.

LBO: Endoscopic stenting may be used for temporary relief in malignant obstructions or preoperatively.

Prognosis:
Delayed intervention, particularly in strangulated or perforated bowel obstruction, significantly increases mortality (up to 30% in complicated cases compared to 3% in uncomplicated SBO).

Controversies and Advances

Diagnostic challenges: Neither clinical signs nor plain radiography reliably identify strangulation. Biomarkers like intestinal fatty acid-binding protein show promise but are not widely available.

Emerging technologies: Improved sensitivity of imaging modalities such as CT and novel biomarkers could revolutionize early detection and management.

References

1. Mizell JS, Turnage RH. Intestinal obstruction. In: Feldman M, Friedman LS, Brandt LJ, editors. Sleisenger and Fordtran's Gastrointestinal and Liver Disease: Pathophysiology, Diagnosis, and Management. 10th ed. Philadelphia: Elsevier/Saunders; 2016. p. 2154–2170.

2. Reddy SR, Cappell MS. Clinical presentation, diagnosis, and management of small bowel obstruction: A systematic review. Current Gastroenterology Reports. 2017;19(6):28.

3. Taylor MR, Lalani N. Small bowel obstruction in adults. Academic Emergency Medicine. 2013;20(6):528–544.

4. van Oudheusden TR, Aerts BA, de Hingh IH, Luyer MD. Diagnostic challenges in adhesive small bowel obstruction. World Journal of Gastroenterology. 2013;19(43):7489–7493.

5. Jaffe T, Thompson WM. Radiographic and CT characteristics of large-bowel obstruction in adults, including differential diagnoses and causes. Radiology. 2015;275(3):651–663.

6. Kameda T, Taniguchi N. The role of point-of-care abdominal ultrasound in emergency and critical care settings. Journal of Intensive Care. 2016;4:53.

7. Paulson EK, Thompson WM. Small bowel obstruction: Diagnostic considerations and clinical red flags. Radiology. 2015;275(2):332–342.

8. Azagury D, Liu RC, Morgan A, Spain DA. A structured, evidence-based approach to small bowel obstruction: Evaluation, decision-making, and management strategies. Journal of Trauma and Acute Care Surgery. 2015;79(4):661–668.

9. Ceresoli M, Coccolini F, Catena F, et al. Diagnostic and therapeutic implications of water-soluble contrast agents in adhesive small bowel obstruction: A systematic review and meta-analysis. American Journal of Surgery. 2016;211(6):1114–1125.

Chapter 5
Herniae

Essentials

1. Early surgical intervention is crucial for symptomatic hernias to prevent potentially fatal complications.

2. Hernias may appear as a reducible mass or progress to complications such as incarceration, strangulation, or intestinal obstruction.

3. Femoral hernias are frequently misdiagnosed and, when complications arise, are linked to significant morbidity.

4. Any hernia presenting with complications requires immediate surgical management.

Detailed Analysis and Overview of Hernias

Introduction

A hernia is the abnormal protrusion of an organ or tissue through a weakened area in the surrounding cavity wall. It typically consists of three components: the hernial aperture (opening), the coverings (usually peritoneum and abdominal wall layers), and the contents, which often include omentum or small intestine. Surgical management of hernias involves the reduction of herniated contents, closure of the defect, and reinforcement using sutures or mesh to prevent recurrence.

While hernias can occur in various locations, this discussion emphasizes the common types, with general principles applicable to less frequent variants.

Aetiology, Pathophysiology, and Clinical Features

Inguinal Hernias

Inguinal hernias are the most prevalent type, accounting for approximately 75% of abdominal wall hernias. The lifetime risk is significantly higher in men (27%) than in women (3%), with an annual incidence of 130 per 100,000 individuals. Urgent repairs, often necessitated by complications, account for up to 9% of cases and are more common in the elderly, where outcomes are associated with higher morbidity.

Direct Inguinal Hernias: These hernias pass directly through the posterior wall of the inguinal canal due to weakened abdominal muscles. They are often bilateral, seen in older adults, and rarely strangulate because of their wide necks.

Indirect Inguinal Hernias: These occur when the hernial sac emerges through the internal inguinal ring, traversing the inguinal canal and possibly descending into the scrotum. The narrow internal ring predisposes to irreducibility and strangulation, making timely diagnosis essential.

Clinical tests can distinguish between direct and indirect hernias. Pressure applied over the internal ring may retain an indirect hernia, while a direct hernia requires broader support to prevent re-protrusion.

Femoral Hernias

Femoral hernias are located lateral and inferior to the pubic symphysis, involving the femoral canal and presenting medial to the femoral vein. They occur more frequently in women, especially the elderly or obese, and tend to complicate early. Due to their subtle presentation, they are often misdiagnosed. Prompt surgical intervention is crucial, as complications such as bowel obstruction can escalate mortality rates to as high as 5% during emergency repairs.

Umbilical Hernias

Common in neonates, umbilical hernias usually resolve by age four. In adults, they may occur around the umbilicus, particularly in obese individuals. Though complications are rare, they can mimic abdominal wall cellulitis when present.

Epigastric Hernias

Epigastric hernias appear in the midline above the umbilicus and often involve entrapped extraperitoneal fat, causing localized pain.

Other Types of Hernias

Obturator Hernias: Rare hernias through the obturator foramen, typically presenting as bowel obstruction in frail elderly women.

Spigelian Hernias: These occur due to defects in the lateral abdominal wall, presenting as reducible lumps, often in elderly males.

Incisional Hernias: Found at previous surgical sites, these result from weakened tissue allowing viscera to protrude.

Sportsman's Hernias: Also known as athletic , these hernias involve posterior inguinal wall weakness without a visible bulge. Ultrasound aids in diagnosis, with surgical repair often necessary for symptom resolution.

Complications

Hernias initially present as reducible masses, but may progress to incarceration, bowel obstruction, or strangulation. Strangulation results in compromised blood flow, leading to ischemia, necrosis, and potential perforation. Richter's hernia, where only a portion of the bowel wall is trapped, presents uniquely with strangulation signs but no obstruction.

Neglected cases may develop fistulas, with bowel contents discharging through the abdominal wall.

Management Strategies

Reduction

Manual reduction is an option for incarcerated hernias without signs of strangulation or obstruction. This procedure requires careful manipulation, adequate analgesia, and vigilance for complications. Reduction alleviates symptoms but should not delay definitive surgical repair.

Surgical Repair

Timely elective repair minimizes the risks of complications. Inguinal hernia repairs are among the most common surgical procedures globally, performed using open or laparoscopic approaches. Laparoscopic methods, though technically challenging, reduce postoperative pain and recovery time but may carry a higher risk of visceral injuries and cost.

Emergent cases, such as those involving obstruction or strangulation, require prompt surgical intervention following adequate fluid resuscitation and stabilization.

Controversies and Challenges

1. Diagnosis and Management of Sportsman's Hernias: Optimal strategies remain debated, particularly regarding the need for surgery.

2. Laparoscopic Versus Open Repair: While minimally invasive techniques are gaining popularity, the associated costs and operator dependency require consideration.

3. Use of Mesh: The choice between synthetic and biological mesh remains contentious, with several products recalled due to safety concerns.

Chapter 6
Gastroenteritis

Essentials

1. Clinical Presentation and Diagnosis
Gastroenteritis is generally a mild, self-limiting condition that is typically diagnosed based on clinical symptoms. It often requires no specific diagnostic tests and resolves naturally with supportive care, including symptomatic management and oral rehydration therapy.

2. Key Symptoms
The hallmark symptom of gastroenteritis is diarrhea, often accompanied by nausea, vomiting, abdominal cramps, lethargy, fever, and varying levels of abdominal discomfort.

3. Clinical Assessment
Physical examination aims to confirm the presence of gastroenteritis, rule out other

potential causes, and evaluate the extent of dehydration.

4. Causative Pathogens

A wide range of infectious agents, including viruses, bacteria, and protozoa, can lead to gastroenteritis.

Viruses: Common pathogens in developed regions include rotavirus and norovirus.

Bacteria: Frequently implicated organisms include Campylobacter , Staphylococcus aureus, Escherichia coli, Shigella , and Salmonella enteritidis.

Protozoa: Giardia lamblia is a notable protozoan cause.

5. Treatment Principles

The cornerstone of treatment includes:

Rehydration: Replenishing fluids orally or via intravenous therapy based on the severity of dehydration.

Symptom Management: Antiemetic agents may be used to alleviate nausea and vomiting.

Targeted Therapy: In specific cases, antimicrobial agents may be necessary to treat bacterial or protozoal infections.

6. Public Health Impact

The introduction of the rotavirus vaccine in 2007 in Australia has significantly reduced the incidence of gastroenteritis caused by both rotavirus and other pathogens, illustrating the importance of vaccination in disease control.

Introduction

Gastroenteritis represents a significant clinical and public health concern worldwide. While its impact varies between regions, it is particularly severe in developing countries where poor water quality and inadequate sanitation contribute to high rates of morbidity and mortality, especially among vulnerable populations such as children and the elderly.

The condition arises from infections in the gastrointestinal tract caused by viruses, bacteria, and protozoa, often transmitted through the fecal-oral route. Symptoms typically include diarrhea, abdominal cramps, nausea, vomiting, lethargy, malaise, and fever. These manifestations vary in severity and duration, lasting anywhere from a single day to over three weeks.

In developed countries, gastroenteritis is less associated with mortality but still causes considerable disruption. It leads to discomfort, loss of productivity, and school absences. Many patients seek emergency care due to the rapid onset of symptoms, severe abdominal pain, frequent diarrhea, or concerns about dehydration.

Pathogenesis and Pathology

The gastrointestinal tract naturally encounters numerous microorganisms daily, but only a small fraction result in clinical illness. The body's defenses include gastric acid, normal bowel flora, bile salts, mucosal immune responses, bowel motility, and secreted immunoglobulin A. Disruption of these defenses—due to conditions like achlorhydria, immunodeficiency, bowel stasis, or antibiotic-induced dysbiosis—can increase susceptibility to infection.

For example, rotavirus infections are more common in children due to a lack of immunity from prior exposure. In contrast, patients with weakened immunity or altered gastrointestinal physiology are at greater risk for severe disease.

Microbiology

Gastroenteritis can result from a wide array of pathogens, including viruses (e.g., rotavirus, norovirus, adenovirus), bacteria (e.g., Escherichia coli, Salmonella, Shigella), and protozoa (e.g., Giardia lamblia, Entamoeba). These organisms employ various mechanisms to induce illness, such as toxin production, direct invasion of the intestinal lining, or a combination of both.

Preformed Toxins: Pathogens like Staphylococcus aureus and Bacillus cereus release toxins in food, which, once ingested, act rapidly to cause vomiting and mild diarrhea.

Invasive Mechanisms: Bacteria such as Shigella and Salmonella invade intestinal mucosa, causing inflammation and cytotoxic damage. Some strains of E. coli, like enterohaemorrhagic E. coli (EHEC), produce toxins that can lead to hemorrhagic colitis and hemolytic uremic syndrome.

Protozoan Infections: Organisms like G. lamblia adhere to the intestinal mucosa, causing inflammation and nutrient malabsorption.

The introduction of vaccines, such as the rotavirus vaccine in Australia, has significantly reduced emergency visits and hospitalizations related to gastroenteritis, including cases not directly caused by rotavirus, highlighting indirect population benefits.

Epidemiology

In Australia, gastroenteritis affects approximately 17.2 million people annually, with 32% of cases being foodborne, leading to around 15,000 hospitalizations and 80 deaths each year. The economic burden on healthcare systems is estimated at $30 million annually. Globally, norovirus is the leading cause of gastroenteritis, responsible for outbreaks in aged care, healthcare, and childcare facilities, underscoring its significant societal impact.

Clinical Features

History

The diagnosis of gastroenteritis is primarily clinical, aiming to confirm the condition, exclude other potential diagnoses, and assess dehydration severity. According to the World Health Organization, gastroenteritis is characterized by three or more loose stools within a 24-hour period. Stool frequency, volume, and characteristics should be assessed, as some pathogens, like E. coli and Shigella, may produce bloody diarrhea, while others, such as Giardia, cause pale, greasy stools.

Other common symptoms include abdominal pain, often described as colicky and diffuse, and vomiting, which is typically transient and associated with toxin-producing organisms.

Systemic signs like fever and lethargy may also occur, particularly in cases involving invasive pathogens.

Physical Examination

A thorough examination focuses on the abdomen and hydration status. Vital signs, including temperature and urine output, are critical in assessing dehydration severity. In mild cases, physical findings are often unremarkable, but severe dehydration may present with tachycardia, hypotension, and reduced skin turgor. Localized abdominal tenderness or peritoneal signs should prompt consideration of alternative diagnoses.

Special Considerations

1. Traveler's Diarrhea: Travelers to regions such as Southeast Asia or Central America are at high risk, with bacteria like enterotoxigenic E. coli being the most common cause. While usually

self-limiting, prophylactic antibiotics are rarely recommended.

2. Immunocompromised Patients: Individuals with weakened immune systems are susceptible to uncommon pathogens, including Cryptosporidium and Cytomegalovirus. These infections are often more severe and require targeted antimicrobial therapy.

3. Hospital-Acquired Diarrhea: Clostridium difficile is the primary cause of antibiotic-associated diarrhea, ranging from mild illness to life-threatening colitis. Prompt diagnosis and treatment are essential to mitigate complications.

Clinical Investigations

In most cases, diagnosing gastroenteritis does not require clinical investigations, nor are they typically essential for effective management. However, identifying the causative agent can be beneficial during outbreaks to implement necessary public health interventions and limit disease transmission. In cases involving prolonged symptoms or specific clinical presentations (e.g., Campylobacter, Giardia, or Salmonella infections), isolating the pathogen can guide antimicrobial therapy or determine carrier status. While patient history and physical examination may provide diagnostic clues, they lack reliability due to overlapping clinical manifestations among different pathogens. Laboratory testing remains the most definitive diagnostic method.

Pathogen identification involves microscopy and culture of stool samples, particularly targeting pathogenic bacteria, ova, cysts, or parasites. Fresh stool specimens are preferred, and multiple samples may be required for organisms that shed intermittently. For rotavirus, antigen detection is achieved via PCR, enzyme-linked immunosorbent assay (ELISA), or latex agglutination.

In dehydrated or systemically unwell patients, laboratory investigations such as full blood count, serum electrolytes, and glucose levels are warranted. In rare cases with signs of systemic illness or suspected sepsis, blood cultures and liver function tests may be necessary. Imaging, such as abdominal X-rays, is reserved for excluding conditions like bowel obstruction or free intra-abdominal gas.

Treatment

The cornerstone of gastroenteritis management includes fluid and electrolyte replacement, symptom alleviation, and selective antimicrobial therapy when indicated.

1. Fluid Replacement:
Fluid loss can be managed orally, via nasogastric tubes, or intravenously, depending on patient cooperation, dehydration severity, rehydration urgency, and comorbid conditions. Oral rehydration solutions (ORS) containing balanced

glucose, sodium, and potassium formulations are most effective, even in resource-limited settings. Commercially available ORS is preferred over high-glucose fluids (e.g., undiluted juices or sodas), which can exacerbate fluid loss through hyperosmolar effects. Caffeinated beverages should also be avoided due to their diarrheagenic potential.

Intravenous rehydration is indicated for patients in shock or with worsening dehydration despite oral fluids. Normal saline is typically initiated, with adjustments for ongoing losses and fluid deficits. Potassium supplementation should be based on serum levels, as hypokalemia indicates significant total body potassium depletion. Transition to oral fluids is recommended as soon as tolerable.

2. Symptom Management:
Antiemetics such as metoclopramide, prochlorperazine, or ondansetron are effective for controlling severe vomiting in adults. Oral ondansetron has also shown utility in pediatric

patients failing initial oral rehydration attempts. Antimotility agents like loperamide can reduce stool frequency and illness duration but are associated with adverse effects and should be reserved for essential cases.

3. Antibiotic Use:
Antibiotics are generally unnecessary in mild gastroenteritis, as most cases are self-limiting. However, persistent diarrhea, fever beyond three days, or severe symptoms may warrant investigation for bacterial causes. Specific antibiotics may be used for:

Giardia: Tinidazole or Metronidazole

Amoebiasis: Metronidazole plus paromomycin

Shigella: Ciprofloxacin, norfloxacin, or co-trimoxazole

Campylobacter: Azithromycin or ciprofloxacin

Salmonella: Antibiotics are reserved for vulnerable groups (e.g., infants, elderly, immunocompromised), with options including azithromycin or ciprofloxacin. Routine antibiotic use in uncomplicated Salmonella is contraindicated as it may prolong the carrier state.

Controversies and Emerging Perspectives

Role of Stool Testing: The necessity of routine stool microscopy and culture remains debated, especially for self-limiting illnesses.

Public Health Surveillance: Emergency departments (EDs) play a critical role in tracking and reporting community gastroenteritis trends.

Assessing Dehydration: The reliability of physical examination alone in evaluating dehydration severity is questioned.

Ondansetron for Rehydration: Evidence supports its role in enhancing oral rehydration therapy, particularly in pediatric cases.

Empirical Antibiotic Therapy: Determining when to initiate empirical antibiotics in severe or atypical presentations requires further clarity.

References

1. Buttery, J. P., Lambert, S. B., Grimwood, K., et al. (2011). Reduction in rotavirus-associated acute gastroenteritis following the inclusion of the rotavirus vaccine in Australia's National Childhood Vaccine Schedule. Pediatric Infectious Disease Journal, 30(Supplement 1), S25–S29.

2. Australian Government Department of Health and Aged Care. Norovirus prevention and control guidelines. Retrieved from the Department of Health website. Accessed in 2018.

3. Cheng, A. C., McDonald, J. R., & Thielman, N. M. (2005). Infectious diarrhea in developed and developing countries. Journal of Clinical Gastroenterology, 39, 1–17.

4. Cheng, A. C., Ferguson, J. K., Richards, M. J., et al. (2011). Australasian Society for Infectious Diseases guidelines for diagnosing and managing Clostridium difficile infections. Medical Journal of Australia, 194, 353–358.

5. Guerrant, R. L., Van Gilder, T., Steiner, S., et al. (2001). Practice guidelines for managing infectious diarrhea. Clinical Infectious Diseases, 32, 331–350.

Chapter 7
Haematemesis and Melaena

Essentials

1. Priority of Resuscitation: Immediate focus should be on resuscitation, emphasizing the restoration of vital organ perfusion through intravascular volume replacement.

2. Role of Upper Gastrointestinal Endoscopy: Early upper GI endoscopy is crucial as it not only serves as a diagnostic tool but often facilitates definitive therapeutic intervention. Prompt endoscopy is recommended whenever feasible.

Introduction

Upper gastrointestinal bleeding (UGIB) is a significant medical emergency associated with notable morbidity and mortality. Despite advancements in drug therapies, endoscopic techniques, interventional radiology, surgical approaches, and supportive care, mortality rates remain approximately 6% to 10%. However, trends in the United Kingdom and the United States suggest a gradual decline in mortality. Currently, fewer than 2% of UGIB cases necessitate emergency surgery. The patient demographic presenting with UGIB is increasingly elderly, with a higher prevalence of comorbid conditions, which likely contributes to the modest improvements in outcomes despite technological advancements. Most fatalities are now attributed to multiple organ failure stemming from pre-existing comorbidities, rather than exsanguination.

Definitions, Epidemiology, and Pathogenesis

UGIB refers to bleeding originating within the gastrointestinal (GI) tract proximal to the ligament of Treitz, whereas bleeding distal to this point is classified as lower GI bleeding. Key clinical presentations include:

Haematemesis: Vomiting bright red blood.

Coffee-ground vomiting: Vomiting of digested blood clots.

Melaena: Passage of black, tarry stools caused by bacterial degradation of hemoglobin in the gut, typically indicating UGIB but occasionally linked to lower GI sources.

Hematochezia: Passage of bright red blood per rectum; in UGIB, this suggests a rapid and significant hemorrhage, doubling the mortality risk.

Peptic ulcer disease remains the leading cause of UGIB, accounting for 36% of cases as per recent

UK audits. This condition is closely linked to Helicobacter pylori (H. pylori) infection, NSAID use (including aspirin), smoking, and alcohol consumption. Additional etiologies include gastroduodenal erosions, oesophagitis (15%), esophagogastric varices (11%-20% in younger patients), Mallory-Weiss tears (<5%), and less common vascular lesions (e.g., angiodysplasia and aortoenteric fistula).

Prevention

Effective management of UGIB involves addressing modifiable risk factors:

1. H. pylori eradication has significantly reduced peptic ulcer disease incidence.

2. NSAID restriction, particularly in elderly patients, remains crucial. Alternatives such as ibuprofen (with a lower GI risk profile) and short-term, low-dose regimens are preferred. For high-risk patients, co-prescription of proton

pump inhibitors (PPIs) is recommended to enhance gastric mucosal protection.

Clinical Features

Initial evaluation should confirm the GI origin of bleeding. Differentiating UGIB from swallowed blood (e.g., from epistaxis) is essential. Key diagnostic considerations include:

History of epigastric pain or dyspepsia: Indicative of peptic ulcer disease, though this may be absent in elderly or NSAID/corticosteroid users.

NSAID use: Doubles the UGIB risk.

Classic nausea and vomiting history: Common in Mallory-Weiss tears.

Alcohol abuse with portal hypertension: Suggestive of varices, though 40% of cirrhotic patients bleed from non-variceal sources.

Stress ulcers: Associated with burns, trauma, head injury, sepsis, and hypotension.

Assessment should also account for comorbid conditions (e.g., chronic renal failure, coagulopathies) and medications (e.g., anticoagulants, antiplatelets). Stool examination, including testing for occult blood, aids in diagnosis and prognostication.

Indicators of bleeding severity include:

Vomitus characteristics: Bright red haematemesis suggests severe bleeding, while coffee-ground vomit indicates slower bleeding.

Stool color: Black tarry stools suggest UGIB; bright red stools suggest brisk bleeding.

Hemodynamic instability and poor response to resuscitation signify significant hemorrhage.

For unstable patients, urgent fluid resuscitation and expedited endoscopy are critical.

Severity Scoring

Severity scoring systems, such as the Rockall and Glasgow-Blatchford scores (GBS), aid in risk stratification:

GBS: Identifies patients suitable for outpatient management, with a score of 0–1 indicating low risk.

Rockall score: Predicts outcomes based on clinical and endoscopic findings.

These tools guide clinical decision-making, including the need for early intervention or hospitalization.

Clinical Investigations

Blood Tests

Routine investigations include full blood count, coagulation studies (e.g., INR/PT), liver function tests, urea, and creatinine levels. Elevated urea relative to creatinine often indicates UGIB. Venous blood gas and lactate levels assess acid-base balance and occult hypoperfusion, respectively.

Imaging

Chest X-rays may be warranted for aspiration risks, suspected perforation, or cardiopulmonary comorbidities, although UGIB-related perforation is rare.

Endoscopy

Endoscopy remains the cornerstone for UGIB diagnosis and management:

1. Diagnostic utility: Provides >90% specificity in identifying bleeding sources.

2. Risk assessment: Endoscopic findings predict rebleeding and mortality, influencing monitoring and outpatient suitability.

3. Therapeutic interventions: Includes sclerotherapy, coagulation techniques, and variceal banding, reducing rebleeding by 75% and mortality by 40% in high-risk peptic ulcers.

Endoscopy should ideally be performed once the patient is hemodynamically stable, with airway protection in place, to maximize safety and effectiveness.

Targeted Therapies for Upper Gastrointestinal Bleeding (UGIB)

Peptic Ulcer Disease (PUD)

Spontaneous Resolution and Mortality: Approximately 80% of bleeding peptic ulcers resolve spontaneously, with a reported mortality rate of 5%–6%, which is significantly lower than that observed in variceal bleeding.

Drug Therapy

1. Acid Suppression and Haemostasis:

The process of haemostasis is influenced by gastric pH levels. Acid suppression has been hypothesized to decrease re-bleeding rates, surgical intervention, and mortality.

2. Histamine (H2) Antagonists:

A 2002 meta-analysis found that H2 antagonists offered limited efficacy. They reduced re-bleeding by 7.2%, surgery by 6.7%, and mortality by 3.2% for gastric ulcers. However, they had no significant effect on duodenal ulcers. Consequently, H2 antagonists are not recommended for contemporary UGIB management.

3. Proton Pump Inhibitors (PPIs):

PPIs remain the cornerstone of PUD management due to their potent and sustained acid suppression.

Guidelines advocate intravenous administration, beginning with a bolus followed by high-dose continuous infusion. While pre-endoscopy PPI use is not routinely supported, it should not delay early endoscopy.

High-risk bleeding ulcers benefit from PPIs, reducing re-bleeding rates within seven days. When intravenous PPIs are unavailable, high-dose oral PPIs (four times the standard dose) are effective.

Addressing reversible risk factors, such as H. pylori infection and NSAID use, is essential for preventing recurrence.

4. Somatostatin and Octreotide:

Although initial studies showed promise, meta-analyses yielded inconsistent results, indicating no mortality benefit. These agents are no longer recommended for acute PUD management.

Endoscopic Therapy

Endoscopy is central to UGIB management, having largely replaced surgery.

Techniques: Combination therapy, including submucosal adrenaline injection with thermal cautery or mechanical clips, is the most effective option for active bleeding ulcers.

Surgical Intervention

Surgery is required in fewer than 2% of cases, typically for intractable or recurrent bleeding, especially in older patients or those with significant comorbidities.

Indications include massive transfusion requirements, refractory shock, or failed endoscopic treatment.

Salvage Surgery: Associated with poorer outcomes, early surgical consultation is advised for high-risk patients.

Trans-Arterial Embolization: Used selectively as an alternative to open surgery, with success rates up to 69%, comparable to surgical outcomes.

Gastro-Oesophageal Varices

While accounting for only 2%–15% of UGIB, gastro-oesophageal variceal bleeding is severe, with spontaneous cessation in only 20%–30% of cases. Mortality rates range from 25%–40%.

Drug Therapy

1. Vasoactive Agents:

Somatostatin and Octreotide: Reduce splanchnic blood flow and portal pressure, achieving haemostasis in 74%–92% of cases.

Vasopressin: Effective in 50%–75% of cases but contraindicated in coronary artery disease due to cardiovascular risks.

Terlipressin: A synthetic vasopressin analogue with a 34% relative mortality risk reduction and fewer side effects, recommended for variceal bleeding.

2. Antibiotic Prophylaxis:

Broad-spectrum antibiotics improve survival in variceal bleeding patients with chronic liver disease. Early intravenous administration (e.g., cephalosporins or quinolones) is advised.

Endoscopic Therapy

1. Esophageal Varices:

Endoscopic Variceal Ligation (EVL) is preferred, offering superior outcomes compared to sclerotherapy, with reduced complications and mortality.

Sclerotherapy is reserved for cases where EVL is not feasible.

2. Gastric Varices:

Cyanoacrylate injection is the treatment of choice, often combined with drug therapy.

Balloon Tamponade

Balloon tamponade provides temporary control for massive or refractory variceal bleeding but has significant limitations:

Complications: Risks include aspiration, esophageal perforation, and re-bleeding upon deflation.

Usage: Reserved as a bridge to definitive interventions, requiring intensive monitoring and skilled staff.

Transjugular Intrahepatic Portosystemic Stent-Shunt (TIPSS)

Procedure: Creates a portosystemic shunt to control bleeding in 90% of cases, offering a less invasive alternative to surgery.

Indications: Recommended for patients with ongoing bleeding despite EVL or sclerotherapy, provided there are no contraindications (e.g., hepatic encephalopathy or severe liver failure).

Surgical Options

With advancements in endoscopic techniques, the role of surgery is limited to refractory cases. Options include shunt surgery and esophageal transection, though survival benefits are uncertain.

Disposition and Risk Stratification

1. Admission Criteria:

ICU or HDU admission is indicated for suspected variceal bleeding, hemodynamic instability, or significant comorbidities.

Elderly patients require lower admission thresholds due to reduced physiological reserves.

2. Outpatient Management:

Selected low-risk patients (e.g., GBS ≤ 2) may be managed as outpatients following early endoscopy, provided there is minimal risk of adverse events.

Chapter 8
Peptic Ulcer Disease Management

Essentials

1. Primary Causes: Helicobacter pylori is implicated in 70% to 90% of peptic ulcer cases, with the majority of the remaining cases linked to the use of non-steroidal anti-inflammatory drugs (NSAIDs).

2. Clinical Presentation: Patients may present with symptoms ranging from mild dyspepsia to severe, life-threatening complications.

3. Diagnostic Approach: Endoscopy remains the gold standard for a definitive diagnosis.

4. Medical Management: The majority of cases can be effectively treated with a combination of antisecretory medications and antibiotics when appropriate.

5. Surgical Intervention: Surgery may become necessary for managing complications such as bleeding, perforation, or gastric outlet obstruction.

6. Radiological Considerations: An erect chest X-ray that appears normal does not rule out the possibility of an ulcer perforation.

7. Related Conditions: Peptic ulcer disease is closely associated with gastritis.

Introduction

Peptic (gastroduodenal) ulcers refer to structural defects in the gastrointestinal lining that extend into the muscularis mucosa. The term "gastritis" denotes inflammation linked to mucosal injury, while "gastropathy" describes epithelial damage and regeneration without accompanying inflammation.

The identification of Helicobacter pylori significantly altered the understanding of peptic ulcer disease's causes and mechanisms. Previously seen as a chronic, recurrent condition, it is now considered treatable and curable. Patients with peptic ulcers may present in emergency settings with classic ulcer symptoms, nonspecific abdominal or chest pain, or severe complications such as perforation or bleeding.

Aetiology, Genetics, Pathogenesis, and Pathology

Aetiology

Peptic ulcer disease (PUD) is primarily associated with H. pylori infection and nonsteroidal anti-inflammatory drug (NSAID) use. Smoking also contributes to disease development, but it does not influence H. pylori recurrence or relapse post-eradication.

Gastritis is typically caused by infections (e.g., H. pylori), autoimmune conditions, or hypersensitivity reactions. Gastropathy, however, often results from irritants such as NSAIDs, alcohol, bile reflux, ischemia, hypovolemia, or chronic congestion.

Genetics

Studies predating H. pylori discovery suggest that PUD may have a genetic predisposition, potentially involving polygenic inheritance. However, the extent to which genetics directly predispose individuals to H. pylori infection remains uncertain.

Pathogenesis and Pathology

H. pylori compromises the mucosal barrier by adhering to the gastric epithelium and releasing enzymes and toxins. This disrupts the mucosa, making it vulnerable to acid damage and triggering an inflammatory response.

NSAIDs contribute to ulcer formation by inhibiting prostaglandin synthesis, leading to increased gastric acid secretion, decreased bicarbonate production, reduced blood flow to the gastric lining, and lower mucosal protective factors. Gastric ulcers are more commonly associated with NSAID use.

Epidemiology

Globally, approximately 50% of the population is infected with H. pylori. Prevalence varies by region due to factors like dietary habits and socioeconomic conditions. Poor hygiene and lower socioeconomic status are linked to higher rates of H. pylori infection.

Most individuals with H. pylori remain asymptomatic, but the bacterium is a significant contributor to peptic ulcer disease. While H. pylori incidence has declined in developed regions, it remains the leading cause of duodenal ulcers and a major cofactor for gastric ulcers. Studies report H. pylori infection in 90%-95% of duodenal ulcers and 70% of gastric ulcers. Eradication significantly reduces ulcer recurrence rates.

NSAIDs also cause gastrointestinal toxicity, with approximately 50% of long-term NSAID users showing endoscopic evidence of ulcers, erosions, or erythema, often without symptoms. Risk factors for NSAID-related ulcer complications include advanced age, prolonged use, high doses, concurrent use of corticosteroids or anticoagulants, and a history of ulcers.
Shorter-acting NSAIDs like ibuprofen are less ulcerogenic than longer-acting ones. Although COX-2 inhibitors (coxibs) reduce ulcer risk compared to traditional NSAIDs, they still carry a higher risk than placebo. Combining coxibs with proton pump inhibitors (PPIs) lowers ulcer risk, though coxibs may hinder healing in existing ulcers. Evidence also suggests a synergistic interaction between H. pylori and NSAIDs in causing ulcers and bleeding.

Other factors like smoking, alcohol, and stress, though less significant since the discovery of H. pylori, may still delay healing and increase ulcer risk. Rare causes include Zollinger-Ellison syndrome.

Clinical Features

History

Peptic ulcers can present with a spectrum of symptoms, with many cases being asymptomatic until complications arise. The most common symptom is epigastric discomfort, often described as a burning or gnawing pain radiating to the chest or back. Accompanying symptoms may include belching, nausea, vomiting, early satiety, and variable responses to food intake. The pain typically fluctuates in intensity, occurring intermittently over time.

However, "indigestion" or "dyspepsia" symptoms lack diagnostic precision for peptic ulcers. Less than 25% of patients with dyspepsia

have confirmed PUD, and many patients with ulcer complications report no prior symptoms. Other presentations include nonspecific abdominal or chest pain, requiring differentiation from conditions like myocardial ischemia, biliary disease, or pancreatitis.
Severe presentations involve complications like acute gastrointestinal bleeding (e.g., hematemesis or melena) or perforation, which manifests as sudden, intense abdominal pain.

Examination

In uncomplicated cases, findings may be limited to epigastric tenderness. Perforations are characterized by severe pain, abdominal rigidity, and signs of peritonitis. Gastrointestinal bleeding often presents as melena on rectal examination.

Differential Diagnosis

The differential diagnosis for upper abdominal pain includes functional dyspepsia (commonest), gastric or pancreatic cancer, biliary disease, pancreatitis, gastroesophageal reflux disease, ischemic bowel disease, and metabolic disorders like hypercalcemia or hyperkalemia.

Clinical Investigations

Laboratory Tests

Blood tests are used to rule out alternative diagnoses and identify complications. Microcytic anemia suggests chronic blood loss, often confirmed by iron studies. Active bleeding may necessitate blood cross-matching and clotting studies, particularly in anticoagulated patients or those with a history of liver disease.

Radiology

While not typically needed for uncomplicated PUD, imaging like erect chest X-rays is critical for suspected perforations. Computed tomography (CT) is the gold standard for detecting pneumoperitoneum. Abdominal X-rays and ultrasounds can help exclude other conditions.

Endoscopy

Endoscopy is the diagnostic tool of choice, providing direct visualization and allowing biopsies for H. pylori testing or malignancy exclusion. Endoscopic interventions can also manage gastrointestinal bleeding.

H. pylori Testing

Diagnostic options include invasive (e.g., biopsy urease testing) and non-invasive (e.g., urea breath tests, stool antigen assays) methods. Non-invasive tests are effective for confirming H. pylori eradication but cannot diagnose PUD directly.

Treatment

Management depends on the cause and presentation. Strategies include eliminating causative factors (e.g., NSAIDs, alcohol), providing symptomatic relief, and addressing H. pylori infection with antibiotics and PPIs. Combined therapies and endoscopic evaluations are essential for persistent symptoms or complications.

Management of NSAID-Induced Ulcers

The American College of Gastroenterology (ACG) guidelines, issued in 2009, emphasize preventive strategies for NSAID-induced ulcer complications. These recommendations highlight the importance of testing for Helicobacter pylori prior to initiating long-term NSAID therapy. Patients testing positive for H. pylori should discontinue NSAIDs whenever clinically feasible and undergo eradication therapy to address the infection.

For patients at moderate risk of ulcer complications and high cardiovascular risk, NSAIDs and COX-2 inhibitors should be avoided, with alternative treatments considered. The primary therapeutic intervention for NSAID-induced ulcers includes an 8-week course of proton pump inhibitors (PPIs) to promote healing and prevent complications.

Surgical Management

Advances in medical therapies have largely restricted the role of surgery in peptic ulcer disease to addressing complications rather than treating the primary condition itself.

Major Complications of Peptic Ulcer Disease

Hemorrhage

Peptic ulcers are a leading cause of upper gastrointestinal (GI) bleeding, occurring in

10%-20% of ulcer cases and accounting for approximately 50% of all upper GI bleeds. Urgent endoscopy is often required for diagnosis and treatment, and in severe cases, surgical intervention may be necessary.

A meta-analysis has shown that acid-reducing agents significantly lower the risk of re-bleeding, though they do not improve mortality rates. Management strategies for hematemesis and melena are explored further in Chapter 7.

Perforation

Peptic ulcer perforation occurs in about 5% of cases, most frequently involving duodenal ulcers (60%), followed by antral (20%) and gastric body ulcers (20%). Approximately one-third to half of perforated ulcers are linked to NSAID use, particularly in elderly individuals.

Clinical Presentation:

Perforations often lead to sudden and severe generalized abdominal pain, with physical examination revealing a rigid abdomen, rebound tenderness, and peritonitis. Delayed presentation, common among elderly or debilitated patients, increases the risk of bacterial peritonitis, sepsis, and shock. Mortality associated with perforations is approximately 5%, with prognosis heavily dependent on timely intervention.

Diagnostic Approach:
Rapid diagnosis is crucial. An erect chest X-ray (CXR) can identify pneumoperitoneum with 70%-80% sensitivity, eliminating the need for further imaging if free air is detected. For equivocal cases, CT or ultrasound may detect smaller amounts of free air or fluid.

Management:
Initial treatment includes fluid resuscitation, close monitoring of renal function via urine output, and empiric antibiotics targeting gram-negative, anaerobic, and enteric flora.

Early administration of intravenous PPIs is essential, alongside adequate analgesia. Surgery, such as a Graham patch repair, is the standard of care after stabilization.
Non-operative management, involving IV fluids, nasogastric suction, antibiotics, and acid suppression, may be an option for patients with rapid spontaneous sealing of the perforation or those deemed unfit for surgery due to comorbidities or delayed presentation.

Penetration

Penetration occurs when a posterior ulcer erodes through the gastric or duodenal wall into adjacent structures, most commonly the pancreas. Unlike free perforation, there is no spillage of luminal contents into the peritoneal cavity.

Clinical Presentation:
Patients report worsening, constant pain radiating to the back that is unresponsive to food

or antacids, accompanied by the loss of pain cyclicity with meals. Serum amylase may be mildly elevated, but clinical pancreatitis is rare.

Diagnosis and Management:
Endoscopy may reveal ulceration, but confirming penetration remains challenging. Management involves addressing the underlying ulcer and mitigating symptoms.

Gastric Outlet Obstruction

This rare complication arises acutely from inflammation and edema at the pylorus or duodenal bulb, or chronically from scarring due to long standing disease.

Prognosis

Peptic ulcer disease carries an excellent prognosis when the underlying cause is identified and treated. Mortality rates are approximately 1 per 100,000 cases, with recent improvements largely attributable to advancements in managing bleeding ulcers through endoscopic therapy and IV PPIs.

Poor Prognostic Factors:

Shock on admission

Renal impairment

Delayed presentation (>12 hours)

Age >70 years

Liver cirrhosis

Immunocompromised states

Perforated gastric ulcers (twice the mortality of duodenal perforations)

Future Directions and Controversies

Potential Developments in the Next 5-10 Years:

1. Development of vaccines for H. pylori to benefit underserved populations.

2. Enhanced understanding and treatment of ulcers unrelated to H. pylori or NSAIDs.

3. Addressing rising antimicrobial resistance in H. pylori.

Ongoing Controversies:

Universal eradication of H. pylori versus targeting symptomatic individuals.

Conservative versus surgical approaches for perforated ulcers.

Interactions between H. pylori infection and low-dose aspirin use.

Disposition

Uncomplicated cases of peptic ulcer disease can often be managed in outpatient settings with appropriate treatment and follow-up.

Here is a paraphrased version of the references you provided:

References

1. Chan FK, Wong VW, Suen BY, et al. Conducted a double-blind, randomized trial to assess the effectiveness of combining a cyclo-oxygenase-2 (COX-2) inhibitor with a proton-pump inhibitor (PPI) in preventing recurrent ulcer bleeding in patients at very high risk. Lancet. 2007;369(9573):1621–1626.

2. Huang JQ, Sridhar S, Hunt RH. Performed a meta-analysis on the role of Helicobacter pylori

infection and non-steroidal anti-inflammatory drugs (NSAIDs) in peptic ulcer disease. Lancet. 2002;359(9300):14–22.

3. Dore MP, Lu H, Graham DY. Investigated the role of bismuth in enhancing the eradication of Helicobacter pylori when combined with triple therapy. Gut. 2016;65(5):870–878.

4. Sachs G, Scott DR. Explored the controversial issue of whether to eradicate or preserve Helicobacter pylori infection. F1000 Med Rep. 2012;4:7.

5. Chey WD, Leontiadis GI, Howden CW, Moss SF. Published a clinical guideline by the American College of Gastroenterology regarding the treatment of Helicobacter pylori infection. Am J Gastroenterol. 2017;112(2):212–239.

6. Lanza FL, Chan FK, Quigley EM. The American College of Gastroenterology's Practice Parameters Committee outlined guidelines for preventing NSAID-related ulcer

complications. Am J Gastroenterol. 2009;104(3):728–738.

7. Melcarne L, García-Iglesias P, Calvet X. Reviewed the management strategies for NSAID-associated peptic ulcer disease. Expert Rev Gastroenterol Hepatol. 2016;10(6):723–733.

8. Zullo A, Hassan C, Campo SM, Morini S. Identified risk factors and preventive strategies for bleeding peptic ulcers in the elderly. Drugs Aging. 2007;24(10):815–828.

Chapter 9
Biliary tract disease

Essentials

1. Gallstones are responsible for over 95% of cases of biliary tract disease.

2. Abdominal pain is the most common symptom in patients with gallbladder disease.

3. Diagnostic tests are primarily aimed at confirming the diagnosis and identifying any complications.

4. The treatment of acute biliary pain (biliary colic) is generally supportive, and patients can often be discharged from the Emergency Department.

5. The treatment of cholecystitis and other gallbladder-related complications involves both supportive care and surgical intervention.

6. Acalculous cholecystitis occurs without the presence of gallstones.

7. Antibiotic therapy is recommended for managing cholangitis and may be necessary for certain patients with cholecystitis.

8. Ultrasound is the preferred imaging modality for most biliary tract disorders.

Introduction

Biliary tract diseases are commonly caused by gallstones, which can lead to a range of complications such as acute or chronic cholecystitis, biliary colic, pancreatitis, cholangitis, and obstructive jaundice. Biliary colic, the most frequent presentation, arises when a gallstone obstructs the cystic duct. The second most common presentation is acute cholecystitis, which occurs when the gallbladder becomes distended, leading to necrosis and ischemia of its mucosal wall. Other conditions of the biliary system include tumors and acalculous cholecystitis, the latter often complicating severe illness. Diagnosis of gallbladder diseases is based on clinical features, laboratory tests, and imaging techniques.

Gallstones and Acute Biliary Pain: Etiology, Genetics, Pathogenesis, and Pathology

The majority of biliary pathologies are due to gallstones. In Western populations, about 80% of gallstones are cholesterol-based, though they can also form from bile pigments due to hemolysis or a mixture of both. When bile becomes concentrated in the gallbladder, crystals may form, which, if trapped in mucus, can grow into sludge and eventually stones. Infection may contribute to stone formation, with bacteria often found inside gallstones. As Lord Moynihan aptly put it, "A gallstone is a tombstone erected to the memory of organisms that lie dead within them." Biliary colic occurs when a gallstone obstructs the cystic duct, causing visceral pain, typically after meals. The stone may eventually dislodge, leading to a temporary relief of symptoms. Persistent obstruction can result in acute cholecystitis, where distension and increased pressure in the gallbladder cause inflammation, ischemia, and mucosal necrosis. Infection is not usually a primary factor in acute cholecystitis, though secondary infection may occur in up to 50% of cases. The hallmark of cholecystitis is ongoing pain, fever, localized peritonism, and an elevated white blood cell count (WCC). Secondary infections are typically caused by aerobic bowel flora, including Escherichia coli and Klebsiella species, and less commonly Enterococcus faecalis. Anaerobic bacteria are rare but may be seen in obstructed cases. Cholangitis requires both biliary obstruction and infection.

Epidemiology

Approximately 10-15% of adults in Western countries have gallstones (cholelithiasis), though the incidence is lower in African and Asian populations. In younger adults, women are affected four times more often than men, but this disparity decreases with age. The lifetime risk for developing gallstones is about 35% in women and 20% in men. Pregnancy and oral contraceptive use increase the risk for women, likely due to hormonal changes that increase cholesterol secretion and bile cholesterol saturation. Other risk factors include aging, diabetes, obesity, rapid weight loss, medications (such as estrogen, octreotide, clofibrate, and ceftriaxone), genetic factors, diseases affecting the terminal ileum, and abnormal lipid profiles.

Two-thirds of gallstones are asymptomatic, and many remain symptom-free for years. The incidence of symptomatic gallstones is low, at 1-4% per year, but increases with factors such as smoking, pregnancy, and obesity. Common complications include biliary colic (56%), acute cholecystitis (36%), and less commonly, pancreatitis or cholangitis. Rare presentations include empyema, perforation, fistula formation, gallstone ileus, hydrops, mucocele, and gallbladder carcinoma.

Prevention

Although several risk factors for gallstones, such as age and gender, are unavoidable, lifestyle modifications may reduce risk. Maintaining a healthy weight and adopting a low-fat, high-fiber diet may help prevent stone formation. Additionally, long-term statin use appears to reduce the risk of gallstones. Ursodeoxycholic acid is beneficial in preventing stones in high-risk patients, such as those undergoing rapid weight loss after bariatric surgery. However, it does not alleviate symptoms once stones have formed.

Clinical Features

History

Biliary colic typically presents as sudden, constant pain in the upper right quadrant (RUQ) or epigastrium, often radiating to the back. Pain generally occurs within a few hours after eating, commonly at night, waking the patient from sleep. The pain typically lasts between one and five hours and may resolve spontaneously or with analgesics. Ongoing pain suggests cholecystitis. Nausea, vomiting, and, in some cases, fever and chills may accompany biliary colic or indicate cholecystitis or cholangitis. Rigors (shivering) are more suggestive of cholangitis.

Examination

The most common finding on physical examination is RUQ tenderness. Vital signs in biliary colic patients are usually normal, and fever is generally absent. The presence of jaundice indicates cholangitis or bile duct obstruction (choledocholithiasis). When pain, jaundice, and high fever with rigors (the Charcot triad) are present, cholangitis should be suspected.

Differential Diagnosis

Differential diagnosis for RUQ pain include:

Peptic ulcer disease, including perforation

Acute pancreatitis

Coronary ischemia, particularly involving the inferior myocardial surface

Appendicitis, especially retrocaecal or in pregnant women

Renal conditions, such as renal colic or pyelonephritis

Colonic disorders, including irritable bowel syndrome

Hepatic diseases, such as hepatitis

Right lower lobe pneumonia

Clinical Investigations

The goal of diagnostic investigations in biliary pain is to confirm the presence of gallstones, assess for complications, and determine the most appropriate treatment approach.

Imaging

Ultrasound: The preferred method for diagnosing gallstones, ultrasound is non-invasive and has a high sensitivity (84%) and specificity (99%). It can confirm the presence of gallstones, measure gallbladder wall thickness, assess the bile duct diameter, and identify fluid collections. However, it is not ideal for detecting stones in the common bile duct (CBD), identifying approximately half of them.

Abdominal X-ray: Plain radiographs are usually not helpful for diagnosing gallbladder disease, but may be useful to rule out other conditions. Only about 10% of gallstones are visible on plain radiographs.

CT Scan: Not typically used as a first-line diagnostic tool, CT is more useful for diagnosing complicated gallbladder diseases, such as acute cholecystitis, gangrene, or perforation. It can also detect bile duct dilation and pneumobilia.

MRI and MRCP: Magnetic resonance imaging, particularly with MRCP, is useful when choledocholithiasis is suspected but not detected on ultrasound.

Blood Tests

Bilirubin and alkaline phosphatase: Levels are generally normal in acute biliary pain but may be mildly elevated in acute cholecystitis.

Amylase/Lipase: Elevated levels help identify pancreatitis, though amylase can also be mildly raised in cholecystitis.

Full blood count: A white blood cell count (WBC) elevation with a left shift is common in cases of cholecystitis and cholangitis. However, up to 40% of patients with these conditions may not show leukocytosis at presentation.

Complications

Gallstone disease can lead to various complications, including:

Cholecystitis

Obstructive jaundice

Cholangitis and sepsis

Gallstone ileus

Gallbladder perforation, particularly in elderly and diabetic patients

Pancreatitis

Treatment

General Measures

Management of biliary colic primarily focuses on pain relief, which can be achieved with oral analgesics, intravenous opioids, or NSAIDs. NSAIDs may be equally effective as opioids, with fewer side effects. There is evidence suggesting that NSAIDs may help prevent the progression of biliary colic to cholecystitis by inhibiting prostaglandin release from the gallbladder wall. Intravenous fluids are recommended for patients with prolonged attacks and vomiting. Additionally, keeping the patient NPO (nothing by mouth) may reduce gallbladder contraction, which helps prevent the release of cholecystokinin.

Antibiotics

Antibiotics are primarily used in the treatment of cholangitis, though their routine use in uncomplicated cholecystitis is debatable. If clinical or radiological signs of infection are present, antibiotics should be administered based on local protocols.

Definitive Care

Cholecystectomy is the definitive treatment for symptomatic gallstones, with a success rate of up to 99%. Laparoscopic cholecystectomy is preferred due to its minimally invasive nature and quicker recovery compared to open surgery. Early cholecystectomy (within 7 days) is recommended for both biliary colic and acute cholecystitis requiring hospitalization. This approach reduces morbidity, operating time, and hospital stay. Non-invasive treatments, such as dissolution therapy and lithotripsy, have limited use, with recurrence rates as high as 50% within 5 years.

Prophylactic cholecystectomy is not recommended for asymptomatic gallstones as the risks of surgery outweigh the benefits. For biliary obstruction, bile duct clearance is also required, which can be performed during cholecystectomy or through endoscopic retrograde cholangiopancreatography (ERCP).

Cholangitis: Pathophysiology, Clinical Features, Investigations, and Management

Pathophysiology

Cholangitis is an infection of the biliary tree, most commonly caused by biliary obstruction. This obstruction can result from choledocholithiasis or from benign or malignant strictures. Infection may also ascend retrogradely through the common bile duct (CBD), often due to procedures like endoscopic retrograde cholangiopancreatography (ERCP). The organisms typically involved are gram-negative bacteria, including Escherichia coli, Klebsiella, Bacteroides, Enterobacter species, enterococci, and group D streptococci. In certain populations, such as those in Asia, cholangitis may be primarily caused by parasitic infections, such as those due to Clonorchis or Opisthorchis .

Clinical Features and Investigations

The classic presentation of cholangitis includes the Charcot triad—jaundice, fever, and right upper quadrant (RUQ) pain. In more severe cases, patients may develop signs of sepsis or septic shock. A white blood cell (WBC) count is typically elevated in these cases. Liver function tests often show a cholestatic pattern of liver injury, and in approximately one-third of patients, serum amylase is elevated. Blood cultures are positive in 20–30% of cases. If biliary fluid is accessible, such as through a drainage procedure, it should be cultured as well.

For diagnosis, transabdominal ultrasonography is the preferred initial imaging modality, as it can detect signs of biliary obstruction or complications like abscess formation. Further imaging studies, such as ERCP, computed tomography (CT) of the biliary tree, or magnetic resonance cholangiopancreatography (MRCP), are used to confirm the diagnosis and assess the extent of the biliary involvement.

Treatment

Patients with cholangitis, especially those presenting with severe sepsis or shock, often require resuscitation. Parenteral antibiotics should be initiated promptly after obtaining blood cultures. Antibiotic therapy should be broad-spectrum, targeting anaerobes and gram-negative bacteria. A commonly used regimen includes amoxicillin 1g IV every 6 hours plus gentamicin 4-6 mg/kg IV daily, although this should be tailored according to local resistance patterns.

Approximately 20% of patients fail to respond to antibiotics or deteriorate rapidly, requiring urgent biliary decompression. This can be achieved through ERCP, either percutaneously or via open surgical decompression.

Controversies in Management

Several issues in the management of cholangitis remain debated, including:

1. The optimal timing of cholecystectomy in patients with choledocholithiasis.

2. The appropriate use of antibiotics in the setting of acute cholecystitis.

3. The best approach to managing choledocholithiasis, particularly in terms of timing and technique for stone extraction.

Conclusion

Cholangitis is a serious condition requiring prompt diagnosis and treatment. Early intervention with appropriate antibiotics and biliary decompression is essential to reduce the risk of complications like sepsis. Ongoing research and clinical debate continue to refine best practices, particularly regarding the timing of surgical interventions and antibiotic stewardship.

Chapter 10
Acute pancreatitis

Introduction

Acute pancreatitis presents two significant challenges: accurate diagnosis and assessment of disease severity. The complexity of diagnosing pancreatitis arises from its non-specific symptoms, which overlap with those of other gastrointestinal disorders. The 2012 revised Atlanta classification for acute pancreatitis defines the condition when two of the following three criteria are met: (1) abdominal pain typical of acute pancreatitis; (2) serum lipase or amylase levels more than three times the normal limit; and (3) characteristic radiological findings on imaging studies such as computed tomography (CT) or magnetic resonance imaging (MRI). Effective patient outcomes depend on early identification of severe pancreatitis. Severe cases require immediate intervention, including intensive care to manage organ failure and to stabilize the patient's condition. After this, the identification of the underlying cause is prioritized, though this may be handled by inpatient teams.

Aetiology and Pathogenesis

The pathogenesis of acute pancreatitis stems from the premature activation of trypsinogen to trypsin, which triggers the release of pancreatic enzymes, leading to pancreatic injury. Approximately 80% of acute pancreatitis cases are mild, characterized by interstitial edema and temporary organ dysfunction that resolves spontaneously. In about 20% of cases, pancreatic necrosis and persistent organ failure occur, with necrotic tissue remaining sterile in 70% of cases and forming a wall, while the remaining 30% may become infected due to the translocation of gut bacteria. This infection triggers a cytokine cascade that can lead to systemic inflammatory response syndrome (SIRS), multi-organ dysfunction syndrome (MODS), and potentially death.

The leading cause of recurrent pancreatitis in males is chronic heavy alcohol consumption (4-5 drinks daily for over five years), which causes both direct toxicity and immune-related effects. Binge drinking without long-term heavy use does not typically induce acute pancreatitis. In females, gallstones are the primary cause of acute pancreatitis. Additional risk factors are listed in the aetiological table, with uncommon causes including hypertriglyceridemia, hypercalcemia, and certain medications (e.g., azathioprine, valproate). In rare cases, trauma, toxins, viral infections, autoimmune diseases, and genetic mutations (such as PRSS1) may contribute to acute pancreatitis.

Epidemiology

The incidence of acute pancreatitis is rising, correlating with increased alcohol consumption and the prevalence of gallstone disease. About 80% of cases are mild and self-limiting, with an overall in-hospital mortality rate of 2%. Key factors influencing mortality include advanced age, obesity, secondary infection, and persistent multi-organ failure.

Clinical Features

Gallstone-induced pancreatitis often presents with sudden, severe epigastric pain radiating to the back. In contrast, pancreatitis caused by other factors, such as alcohol, may develop more gradually and the pain may be less localized. Nausea and vomiting typically accompany the pain. Abdominal tenderness is common, but guarding and rebound tenderness are unusual. Rare signs, such as Cullen's sign (ecchymosis around the umbilicus), Grey Turner's sign (ecchymosis in the flanks), and Fox's sign (ecchymosis in the inguinal region), may indicate retroperitoneal bleeding and appear 36-72 hours after pain onset. Severe pancreatitis is often associated with tachycardia, hypotension, abdominal distension, and shallow breathing due to diaphragmatic irritation and pleural effusion.

Differential Diagnosis

The primary differential diagnoses to consider include perforated viscus, ischemic colitis, leaking abdominal aortic aneurysm, and myocardial ischemia.

Clinical Investigations

Biochemical Tests

Amylase levels typically rise within 2 to 12 hours and normalize in about a week. However, in about 10% of cases, amylase may be falsely normal due to depleted acinar cell mass. False positives may also arise from salivary gland disorders, macroamylasemia, certain cancers, or impaired renal clearance in chronic renal failure. Lipase, which rises within 4 to 8 hours and normalizes in 1 to 2 weeks, is more specific and sensitive than amylase. Serum lipase or amylase levels greater than three times the normal limit are diagnostic for acute pancreatitis, but peak enzyme levels do not correlate with disease severity. For suspected gallstone pancreatitis, alanine aminotransferase (ALT) levels ≥150 IU/L are highly specific (96%) but less sensitive (48%).

Other biochemical markers, such as hematocrit, urea, and creatinine, are useful for monitoring disease progression. C-reactive protein, lactate dehydrogenase, blood gas analysis, calcium, and procalcitonin are also employed to assess severity.

Imaging Studies

In cases where clinical or biochemical data are inconclusive, contrast-enhanced CT scans are the preferred imaging modality, as they can confirm the diagnosis, differentiate from other conditions, assess disease severity, and identify complications. Ultrasound may show gallstones or a dilated bile duct, hinting at gallstone pancreatitis, but is limited by its inability to clearly visualize the pancreas in 25-50% of cases. Magnetic resonance cholangiopancreatography (MRCP) provides a non-invasive alternative to CT with lower nephrotoxicity risk and superior ability to identify complications such as fluid collections, abscesses, or pseudocysts. Plain radiographs offer limited diagnostic utility but may reveal signs such as pleural effusion or calcifications indicative of chronic pancreatitis or infection.

Severe Pancreatitis Scoring Systems

Severe pancreatitis is defined as persistent organ failure lasting more than 48 hours. Several scoring systems have been developed to predict the severity and mortality risk associated with acute pancreatitis, incorporating clinical, laboratory, and radiological data. These systems include:

Ranson's Score: Measures various parameters at admission and 48 hours after onset. A score ≥3 indicates severe pancreatitis.

Modified Glasgow Score: Similar to Ranson's but based on 48-hour parameters.

APACHE II: An assessment of physiological parameters within the first 24 hours.

BISAP Score: Uses early data such as urea levels and mental status changes.

CT Severity Index (Balthazar): Evaluates CT findings of pancreatic inflammation and necrosis.

Treatment

The management of acute pancreatitis is largely supportive, with an emphasis on fluid resuscitation, respiratory support, and pain management:

Oxygen supplementation: Used for patients showing signs of hypoxia, which may suggest ARDS or pleural effusion.

Fluid resuscitation: Critical for replacing third-space fluid losses. Intravenous crystalloids should be administered early, with adjustments based on blood pressure and urine output.

Pain management: Intravenous opioids, such as morphine or fentanyl, are commonly used for pain relief. There is no conclusive evidence linking morphine use to sphincter of Oddi spasm.

Other supportive measures include:

Antibiotics: Reserved for patients with documented infections (e.g., pancreatic abscesses).

Nutritional support: Early enteral feeding is preferred over total parenteral nutrition, especially in severe cases, to support gut function and prevent complications like mucosal atrophy.

Surgical intervention: Infected pancreatic necrosis may require debridement, but this is generally delayed for 4 weeks to allow for proper encapsulation of the necrotic tissue. For stable patients, minimally invasive drainage may be considered.

Chronic pancreatitis

Introduction

Chronic pancreatitis typically presents with recurrent abdominal pain, often radiating to the back. This pain can be exacerbated after eating, leading to a reduced appetite and resulting in weight loss. In some cases, patients may experience symptoms of pancreatic exocrine insufficiency, such as steatorrhea, or endocrine insufficiency, which can manifest as diabetes mellitus. Physical examination may reveal a mass in the epigastrium, potentially indicating the presence of a pseudocyst. Additionally, patients may adopt a characteristic posture to alleviate pain, typically lying on their side with their knees drawn up to their chest.

Aetiology and Pathogenesis

Chronic pancreatitis is commonly attributed to metabolic factors, with excessive alcohol consumption responsible for 60% to 90% of cases. The underlying process involves chronic, irreversible inflammation of the pancreas, leading to fibrosis and calcification. This damage affects both the exocrine and endocrine functions of the pancreas, contributing to the development of pancreatic insufficiency.

Clinical Investigations

Unlike acute pancreatitis, serum amylase and lipase levels are often only mildly elevated or can even be normal in chronic pancreatitis, particularly if the pancreatic gland has undergone atrophy. Endoscopic retrograde cholangiopancreatography (ERCP) remains the gold standard for diagnosing chronic pancreatitis, allowing for detailed imaging of the pancreatic ducts. Non-invasive alternatives, such as contrast-enhanced CT and magnetic resonance cholangiopancreatography (MRCP), offer valuable insights into pancreatic parenchymal changes and the extent of the disease.

Treatment

Managing chronic pancreatitis involves several key considerations:

Alcohol cessation: Continued alcohol use increases the risk of painful flare-ups and accelerates pancreatic dysfunction. Stopping alcohol consumption may require a multidisciplinary approach, including counseling and psychiatric support for cognitive therapy and behavioral modification.

Pain management: Chronic pain is a significant challenge in the management of chronic pancreatitis. Many patients develop chronic pain syndrome, which may lead to opioid dependency. Pain management should be a priority during acute episodes, and early referral to a pain management specialist is recommended to prevent or address opioid misuse. Temporary relief can be achieved through CT-guided celiac ganglion blockade.

Malabsorption: Management of malabsorption includes a low-fat diet and supplementation of pancreatic enzymes, fat-soluble vitamins, and vitamin B12 to address exocrine pancreatic insufficiency. Endocrine insufficiency, often resulting in diabetes mellitus, may necessitate insulin therapy.

Mechanical obstruction: Obstructions can be relieved through endoscopic procedures, surgical resection, or drainage to restore proper pancreatic function.

Controversies in Acute Pancreatitis

Severity Scoring Systems: While multiple scoring systems exist for assessing the severity of acute pancreatitis, none are entirely reliable.

However, they still provide more accurate predictions than clinical judgment alone in identifying cases of severe pancreatitis.

Adipokines and Severe Acute Pancreatitis: The role of adipokines in identifying severe acute pancreatitis remains an area of active research. Understanding their involvement could lead to more precise diagnostic tools for severity assessment.

Hemofiltration in Management: The utility of hemofiltration in treating severe acute pancreatitis is still debated. Its effectiveness in improving patient outcomes requires further investigation to clarify its role in the treatment protocol.

Sphincter of Oddi Dysfunction and Pancreas Divisum: The contributions of sphincter of Oddi dysfunction and pancreas divisum to the development of acute pancreatitis are not fully understood. Their involvement in the pathophysiology of acute pancreatitis remains controversial.

References

1. Banks PA, Bollen TL, Dervenis C, et al. Classification of acute pancreatitis—2012: revision of the Atlanta classification and definitions by international consensus. Gut. 2013;62:102–111.

2. Forsmark CE, Vege SS, Wilcox CM. Acute pancreatitis. N Engl J Med. 2016;375:1972–1981.

3. Phillip V, Huber W, Hagemes F, et al. Incidence of acute pancreatitis does not increase during Oktoberfest, but is higher than previously described in Germany. Clin Gastroenterol Hepatol. 2011;9(11):995–1000.e3.

4. Wu BU. Prognosis in acute pancreatitis. Can Med Assoc J. 2011;183(6):673–677. https://doi.org/10.1503/cmaj.101433.

5. Balthazer EJ. Acute pancreatitis: assessment of severity with clinical and CT evaluation. Radiology. 2002;223:603–613.

6. Khanna AK, Meher S, Prakash S, et al. Comparison of Ranson, Glasgow, MOSS, SIRS, BISAP, APACHE-II, CTSI Scores, IL-6, CRP, and Procalcitonin in Predicting Severity, Organ Failure, Pancreatic Necrosis, and Mortality in Acute Pancreatitis. HPB Surgery. 2013;2013:10. Article ID 367581. https://doi.org/10.1155/2013/367581.

7. Gao W, Yang HX, Ma CE. The value of BISAP score for predicting mortality and severity in acute pancreatitis: a systematic review and meta-analysis. PLOS ONE. 2015;10(6):e0130412. https://doi.org/10.1371/journal.pone.0130412.

8. Harrison DA, D'Amico G, Singer M. The Pancreatitis Outcome Prediction (POP) score: a new prognostic index for patients with severe acute pancreatitis. Crit Care Med. 2007;35:1703–170.

Chapter 11
Acute Appendicitis

Essentials

1. Most Common Cause of Abdominal Pain: Appendicitis is the leading cause of acute abdominal pain that necessitates surgical intervention.

2. Clinical Diagnosis: While the diagnosis is primarily based on clinical evaluation, the absence of a specific diagnostic sign or definitive first-line test can complicate diagnosis.

3. Consequences of Diagnostic Delay: A delay in diagnosis is the main contributor to complications and fatalities and remains a significant cause of medical malpractice claims in emergency care settings.

4. Role of Imaging: Advanced imaging techniques improve diagnostic accuracy and help decrease unnecessary laparotomies. However, computed tomography (CT) should be used selectively to minimize radiation exposure.

5. Surgical Referral and Non-Operative Management: Referral for surgery is warranted when appendicitis is confirmed or strongly suspected. However, non-operative management is becoming increasingly recognized as a viable option for uncomplicated cases.

Introduction

Appendicitis is the leading cause of acute abdominal pain that necessitates surgical intervention and is the most common non-obstetric surgical emergency during pregnancy. While the incidence of appendicitis has decreased in industrialized countries since the late 1940s, it is rising in newly industrialized nations. Appendicitis predominantly affects individuals in their second and third decades of life, with a higher incidence in males (male-to-female ratio of 1.4:1). The overall incidence is approximately 1.9 cases per 1,000 persons annually, and individuals have a lifetime risk of 7%. Diagnostic delays are more common in infants, young children, women of reproductive age, and the elderly. Early diagnosis is critical to prevent complications such as appendiceal perforation, intra-abdominal sepsis, abscess formation, and generalized peritonitis.

Aetiology, Pathogenesis, and Pathology

Appendicitis is often preceded by a bacterial or viral infection in the colon, which leads to mucosal ulceration in the appendix and subsequent bacterial invasion by normal colonic flora. In some cases, luminal obstruction of the appendix occurs due to factors such as fecaliths, lymphoid hyperplasia, parasites, strictures, adhesions, foreign bodies, tumors (e.g., carcinoid or cecal carcinoma), or Crohn's disease. This obstruction causes increased intraluminal pressure, leading to luminal distension and blockage of lymphatic and venous outflow, as well as arterial occlusion, fostering bacterial overgrowth. Inflammation of the serosa leads to irritation of the parietal peritoneum, and in some cases, appendiceal perforation can occur due to high intraluminal pressure.

Clinical Features

Appendicitis is primarily diagnosed clinically, although the presentation can sometimes be atypical, requiring close observation or imaging to confirm the diagnosis. When assessing a patient with acute abdominal pain in the emergency department, it is crucial to consider whether appendicitis could be the underlying cause.

History

The classic presentation of acute appendicitis involves the development of upper midline or periumbilical pain (seen in 70% of cases), which represents visceral pain due to distension of the appendix. This pain progresses over a period of 12-24 hours to the right lower quadrant, which signifies somatic pain caused by irritation of the parietal peritoneum. The migratory nature of the pain is the most characteristic symptom of appendicitis. Associated symptoms often include nausea, anorexia, and vomiting. A low-grade fever (typically between 37.5°C and 38.0°C) is commonly present. Once the pain localizes to the right lower quadrant, it becomes persistent and worsens with movement, deep inspiration, and coughing. Pelvic appendicitis may present with urinary symptoms such as dysuria or frequent urination, or with diarrhea. Atypical presentations may occur if the appendix is located in unusual positions, such as the right upper quadrant (often due to a retrocecal appendix) or left lower quadrant (as seen with a pelvic appendix or situs inversus).

Examination

Examination findings depend on the stage of appendicitis. Vital signs are usually normal, but mild tachycardia and low-grade fever are common. Facial flushing, halitosis, and a dry tongue may be observed. The hallmark physical finding is localized tenderness in the right lower quadrant, with maximal tenderness at McBurney's point (located two-thirds of the way from the umbilicus to the anterior superior iliac spine). This is often accompanied by involuntary muscle guarding and reduced respiratory movement. In obese, elderly, or pediatric patients, or in cases with atypical appendix locations, eliciting guarding may be challenging. Rebound tenderness, a sign of peritoneal irritation, can be assessed by having the patient inhale deeply, cough, or percuss the abdomen. Pain in the right lower quadrant may also be provoked by pressure on the left lower quadrant (Rovsing's sign), and the affected area may exhibit hyperesthesia (Sherren's sign).

Only about 50-70% of patients with acute appendicitis exhibit the classic symptoms and signs. Therefore, additional clinical signs may be helpful, especially when the appendix is in an atypical location. For example, retrocecal appendicitis may irritate the psoas muscle, leading to a positive psoas sign (pain and resistance on passive extension of the right hip). Similarly, a pelvic appendix can cause irritation of the obturator internus muscle, producing a positive obturator sign (pain during passive internal rotation of the right hip). In approximately 10-15% of cases, an abdominal mass may be palpable, indicating inflamed omentum and adherent bowel loops due to a perforated appendix. Recurrent appendicitis is possible even in patients who have undergone previous appendectomy.

In elderly patients, rectal examination may help identify tenderness in the right lateral rectal wall or diagnose a pelvic abscess if a ruptured pelvic appendix is suspected.

Perforation

If the appendicitis has progressed for more than 24 hours, the patient may show signs of perforation, including higher fever (above 38°C) and an elevated white blood cell count greater than 15,000/mm³.

Differential Diagnosis

Appendicitis can mimic a variety of acute abdominal conditions, and it should be considered in any patient presenting with acute abdominal symptoms. Many conditions, such as gastroenteritis, ovarian torsion, ectopic pregnancy, and Crohn’s disease, can present similarly to appendicitis. In some cases, a definitive diagnosis may only be possible during surgery or laparoscopy. However, diagnostic delay can lead to complications such as perforation, abscess formation, or generalized peritonitis, which may result in wound infections, sepsis, or even death.

Clinical Investigations

Urinalysis

A urine dipstick examination is recommended for all patients to rule out urinary tract infections. Pyuria or microscopic hematuria may also be present in cases of appendicitis, but these findings are not specific.

Blood Tests

White blood cell count (WBC) and C-reactive protein (CRP) levels can be useful but are not definitive. A raised WBC count may suggest an acute infection but lacks the specificity to confirm appendicitis. In some patients, particularly infants, the elderly, and pregnant women, the white blood cell response may be reduced or absent. Similarly, normal CRP levels do not exclude appendicitis, although elevated levels combined with an increased WBC count strongly support the diagnosis.

Imaging

Plain abdominal X-rays have low sensitivity and specificity for appendicitis and are rarely helpful in diagnosis. If an X-ray is performed, the presence of a fecalith in the right lower quadrant may support the diagnosis.

Ultrasound is often the preferred first-line imaging modality, particularly in children and as a preliminary step in adults before a CT scan. The appendix can be visualized on ultrasound as a non-compressible, hypoechoic, tubular structure measuring more than 6 mm in diameter, with a thickened wall and possible appendicolith. Color Doppler ultrasound may also show increased vascularity in the appendiceal wall. A normal appendix seen on ultrasound generally rules out appendicitis.

Computed tomography (CT) is highly effective in diagnosing appendicitis, especially in older patients or cases with ambiguous presentations. CT scans show an enlarged, thickened appendix with signs of inflammation, such as periappendiceal fat stranding. Sensitivity and specificity for appendicitis can exceed 98% with the use of contrast-enhanced imaging.

Magnetic resonance imaging (MRI) is recommended for pregnant patients, as it does not involve ionizing radiation. MRI findings of acute appendicitis include an enlarged appendix, fluid-filled lumen, and periappendiceal fat stranding.

Controversies

The application of ultrasound as a first-line diagnostic tool, particularly in adult patients.

The role of conservative management in cases of uncomplicated acute appendicitis.

The utility of laparoscopy in both the diagnosis and treatment of various conditions.

Conclusion

Appendicitis remains a critical condition requiring prompt diagnosis and intervention. The clinical features, laboratory findings, and imaging studies play a vital role in making an accurate diagnosis. Though the condition presents with typical signs in many cases, the clinical picture may vary depending on factors such as age, sex, and anatomical variations. Early recognition is crucial to prevent severe complications, including perforation and peritonitis.

Chapter 12
Inflammatory bowel disease

Essentials

1. The two primary types of inflammatory bowel disease (IBD) are Crohn's disease and ulcerative colitis, with diarrhea and/or abdominal pain being the key clinical symptoms.

2. IBD is a chronic, relapsing condition. Patients may present to the emergency department due to increased disease activity or complications arising from the disease or its treatment.

3. Gastrointestinal complications associated with IBD include dehydration, bleeding, strictures, obstruction, fistulas, sepsis, perforation, neoplasia, and toxic megacolon.

4. Extraintestinal manifestations of IBD commonly include acute arthropathy and skin rashes.

5. Medication-related complications may involve opportunistic infections, particularly in patients taking corticosteroids, immunomodulators, or biological therapies.

6. Patients with moderate to severe IBD typically require hospitalization and specialist consultation, usually from gastroenterology.

7. Initial management for most patients includes medical treatment with aminosalicylates and/or corticosteroids; however, those with intra-abdominal sepsis, perforation, obstruction, or toxic megacolon are more likely to need emergency surgery.

Introduction and Pathology

Inflammatory bowel disease (IBD) encompasses Crohn's disease (CD), ulcerative colitis (UC), and IBD Unclassified (IBD-U), which displays characteristics of both conditions. These are chronic inflammatory disorders of the gastrointestinal (GI) tract caused by an abnormal, persistent inflammatory response. This response is influenced by a combination of genetic, infectious, and environmental factors that disrupt the normal function of intestinal immunity, leading to GI tract injury.

Pathologically, CD and UC differ in their presentation. CD is characterized by patchy transmural inflammation that can affect any part of the GI tract, although ileocolonic involvement is most common. CD is often associated with complications such as fistulas, abscesses, strictures, and obstructions. UC, on the other hand, presents as a continuous, diffuse inflammation confined to the colonic mucosa, typically resulting in bleeding. Clinical manifestations depend on the type and location of the disease. In emergency settings, it is crucial to assess the disease's activity and identify potential complications associated with the disease or its treatment.

Clinical Features

History

UC: The hallmark symptom is bloody diarrhea, which is often accompanied by colicky abdominal pain, urgency, and tenesmus.

CD: Symptoms typically include abdominal pain, anal complaints (such as fissures), diarrhea (without rectal bleeding), and weight loss. Abdominal pain in CD is often localized to the right side and may worsen with eating. In contrast, UC pain is usually less frequent, crampy, located in the lower abdomen, and relieved by defecation. If pain becomes more intense, other GI complications should be considered.

It's important to assess for any extra-intestinal manifestations of IBD, such as arthritis, rashes, and other severe complications like thromboembolism, ocular issues, and hepatobiliary conditions, which require specialized treatment. The risk of venous thromboembolism is notably elevated, especially during disease flare-ups or corticosteroid therapy.

A thorough drug history is essential since medications like aminosalicylates, steroids, immunomodulators (e.g., methotrexate, azathioprine), and biologics (e.g., infliximab, adalimumab) can contribute to IBD complications. In patients on immunosuppressive treatments, it's crucial to screen for sepsis and opportunistic infections. Additionally, biologic agents may increase the risk of hypersensitivity reactions, cancers (e.g., lymphoma), and reactivation of infections such as tuberculosis or viral illnesses.

Smoking significantly worsens CD, so cessation advice should be given to affected patients.

Examination

On physical examination, the abdomen is typically mildly tender without peritonitis. Signs of dehydration or sepsis should be investigated. The presence of fever, dehydration, orthostatic hypotension, abdominal tenderness, distension, and hypoactive bowel sounds may indicate fulminant colitis. Severe abdominal distension raises concerns for toxic megacolon or obstruction. Toxic megacolon, a rare but life-threatening complication of severe colitis, requires immediate intervention. A rectal exam may reveal anal fissures, abscesses, or fistulae, which are more commonly associated with CD.

Investigations

Blood Tests

Full blood count: Assesses anemia and the need for transfusion.

Leukocytosis: Common in acute disease; however, leukopenia may occur in patients on immunosuppressive therapy.

ESR and C-reactive protein: These markers are used to monitor inflammation.

Electrolytes and renal function: Abnormalities may indicate dehydration.

Iron, folate, vitamin B12 deficiencies, and hypoalbuminemia: These are common in IBD.

Liver function tests and elevated amylase/lipase may suggest hepatobiliary issues or drug toxicity.

Fecal Testing

Fecal calprotectin is a highly sensitive non-invasive marker of intestinal inflammation and can be used for monitoring disease activity, detecting relapses, and assessing mucosal healing.

C. difficile testing is critical since this infection is more prevalent in IBD patients and can worsen outcomes.

Cytomegalovirus (CMV) testing is recommended for severe colitis, particularly for patients on immunosuppressants, as CMV colitis is associated with poor prognosis.

Imaging Studies

For acute abdominal pain, abdominal and chest x-rays are useful to detect free gas (which suggests perforation), dilated bowel loops (indicating obstruction), or signs of toxic megacolon (a colon diameter greater than 5.5 cm). MRI and ultrasound are preferred, especially in younger patients, as they expose the patient to less radiation compared to CT. MRI is particularly useful for assessing perineal fistulas. CT is more commonly used in acute scenarios to evaluate complications like obstruction or sepsis. Ultrasound can detect extra-intestinal complications such as gallstones or kidney stones.

Endoscopy

Endoscopy remains the gold standard for diagnosing IBD and assessing disease activity. It is essential for evaluating the presence of strictures or cancer. However, in cases of severe IBD, sigmoidoscopy or colonoscopy should be performed cautiously to avoid the risk of perforation. Capsule endoscopy is not commonly used in acute settings since it offers no additional benefit over cross-sectional imaging.

Severity Assessment

Crohn's Disease Activity Index (CDAI): Though not routinely used in clinical practice, the CDAI uses criteria such as stool frequency, abdominal pain, general well-being, and weight loss to gauge disease severity. A score greater than 450 indicates severe disease.

Ulcerative Colitis: Severity is often determined using the Truelove and Witts criteria, where severe UC is defined by symptoms such as more than six bloody stools daily, elevated heart rate, fever, anemia, and a high ESR.

Gastrointestinal Complications

Toxic Megacolon: This is a life-threatening complication characterized by colonic dilatation ($\geq$5.5 cm) associated with systemic toxicity. Factors such as hypokalemia, hypomagnesemia, and the use of antidiarrheal agents or bowel preparations increase the risk. Early recognition in the emergency department (ED) is critical for successful management, which includes both medical and surgical interventions. If medical management fails, a colectomy may be necessary.

Bowel Perforation: Perforation can occur without toxic megacolon, requiring early detection and surgical consultation.

Strictures and Obstruction: In UC, strictures suggest malignancy until proven otherwise. In CD, strictures may result from acute inflammation, edema, or fibrosis.

Hemorrhage: This is more common in UC due to ulceration of the GI tract.

Fistulae and Abscesses: Fistulae, especially those connecting to the urinary tract or vagina, can cause recurrent infections and other complications.

Infectious Colitis: Both UC and CD patients are prone to superimposed infections, particularly C. difficile.

IBD patients also have an increased risk of developing colon cancer, especially with extensive and prolonged disease.

Treatment

General Management

In the ED, priority should be given to identifying and managing life-threatening complications such as septic shock, severe anemia, or dehydration. After stabilizing the patient, focus should shift to assessing disease activity and identifying complications. Intravenous fluids, correction of electrolyte imbalances, and blood transfusions may be required. Paracetamol and codeine are preferred for managing pain, as stronger opioids are linked to increased mortality in IBD patients.

Medical Therapy

Aminosalicylates: Effective in maintaining remission in UC and small bowel CD.

Corticosteroids: Used for inducing remission, especially in acute flares, but not suitable for long-term maintenance. Prednisone is commonly prescribed, with the dosage gradually reduced.

Biologic Agents: Used for moderate to severe disease, particularly when other treatments are ineffective.

Surgical intervention is indicated for complications such as bowel perforation, obstruction, or toxic megacolon.

Conclusion

The management of IBD requires a comprehensive approach involving timely diagnosis, careful monitoring of disease activity, and appropriate treatment to prevent complications. While most patients can be managed conservatively, severe cases may require urgent surgical intervention. Understanding the pathophysiology, clinical features, and complications of IBD is crucial for effective patient care in both the emergency and long-term settings.

References

1. Gastroenterological Society of Australia. Clinical Update for General Practitioners and Physicians – Inflammatory Bowel Disease, 4th ed. 2017. Available from: http://www.gesa.org.au/resources/clinical-guidelines-and-updates/inflammatory-bowel-disease/.

2. Sairenji T, Collins KL, Evans DV. An overview of inflammatory bowel disease. Prim Care. 2017;44(4):673-692.

3. Torres J, Mehandru S, Colombel JF, Peyrin-Biroulet L. Crohn's disease. Lancet. 2017;389(10080):1741-1755.

4. Ungaro R, Mehandru S, Allen PB, Peyrin-Biroulet L, Colombel JF. Ulcerative colitis. Lancet. 2017;389(10080):1756-1770.

5. Gomollon F, Dignass A, Annese V, et al. Third European evidence-based consensus on the diagnosis and management of Crohn's disease 2016: Part 1—Diagnosis and medical management. J Crohn's Colitis. 2017;11(1):3-25.

6. Magro F, Gionchetti P, Eliakim R, et al. Third European evidence-based consensus on diagnosis and management of ulcerative colitis. Part 1: Definitions, diagnosis, extra-intestinal manifestations, pregnancy, cancer surveillance, surgery, and ileo-anal pouch disorders. J Crohn's Colitis. 2017;11(6):649-670.

7. Bernstein CN, Eliakim A, Fedail S, et al. World Gastroenterology Organisation global guidelines for inflammatory bowel disease: Update August 2015. J Clin Gastroenterol. 2016;50(10):803-818.

8. Harbord M, Eliakim R, Bettenworth D, et al. Third European evidence-based consensus on diagnosis and management of ulcerative colitis. Part 2: Current management. J Crohn's Colitis. 2017;11(7):769-784.

9. Peyrin-Biroulet L, Panes J, Sandborn WJ, et al. Defining disease severity in inflammatory bowel diseases: Current and future directions. Clin Gastroenterol Hepatol. 2016;14(3):348-354.e17.

10. CDAI Calculator: IBD Support Australia. 2012. [cited January 25, 2018]. Available from: https://www.ibdsupport.org.au/cdai-calculator.

11. Mowat C, Cole A, Windsor A, et al. Guidelines for the management of inflammatory bowel disease in adults. Gut. 2011;60(5):571-607.

Chapter 13
Acute Liver Failure (ALF)

Essentials

1. The diagnosis of acute liver failure (ALF) is confirmed when there is a combination of worsening coagulopathy, hepatic encephalopathy, and escalating jaundice.

2. In low- and middle-income countries, viral infections are the leading cause of ALF, with hepatitis E being a significant contributor in many regions.

3. In high-income countries, drug-induced liver injury (DILI) is the primary cause, with paracetamol (acetaminophen) often being the culprit.

4. ALF should be suspected in any patient presenting with recent onset of liver dysfunction, characterized by a prolonged prothrombin time

or an elevated international normalized ratio (INR).

5. Early recognition of ALF is critical, as it allows for the use of antidotes when a reversible cause is identified.

6. The management of ALF involves standard intensive care, along with targeted interventions to identify and mitigate the cause of liver injury. Supportive organ care aims to optimize liver regeneration and restore pre-existing liver function, while simultaneously preventing potential complications.

7. The advent of emergency liver transplantation has significantly improved survival outcomes for ALF patients.

8. Public health initiatives to regulate drug use and reduce the prevalence of hepatotropic viral infections could greatly lower the morbidity and mortality associated with ALF in the future.

Introduction

Acute liver failure (ALF) represents a critical medical emergency, characterized by rapid liver dysfunction leading to altered mental status and coagulopathy in patients who were previously healthy. Its incidence is relatively rare, ranging from one to six cases per million individuals annually in developed countries. The leading causes of ALF include viral hepatitis, drug-induced liver injury (DILI), autoimmune diseases, and shock or hypo-perfusion. Approximately 20% of ALF cases remain of indeterminate origin. The condition primarily affects younger populations, resulting in high rates of morbidity and mortality. ALF is a common indication for emergency liver transplantation, and prior to the availability of transplants, mortality rates exceeded 90%. Multiorgan failure, hemorrhage, infection, and cerebral edema were the leading causes of death. However, with advances in treatment, particularly liver transplantation, 1-year survival rates now exceed 80%. ALF remains an area with limited research, mostly conducted in large centers or through collaborative networks like the NIH-funded Acute Liver Failure Study Group (ALFSG).

Aetiology, Pathogenesis, and Pathology

ALF occurs when hepatocyte death outpaces regeneration, due to various insults leading to either apoptosis or necrosis. Apoptosis is marked by nuclear shrinkage without cell membrane rupture, meaning that intracellular contents are not released, and secondary inflammation does not follow. Conversely, necrosis is associated with ATP depletion, leading to cell swelling and rupture, which releases intracellular contents and triggers inflammation. Causes like paracetamol toxicity primarily result in apoptosis, while ischemia leads to necrosis. The consequence of this cellular damage is rapid progression to coma and death from multiorgan failure.

Epidemiology

The incidence of ALF varies globally, with substantial differences in etiology. In the UK, ALF is responsible for fewer than 500 deaths annually and less than 15% of liver transplants each year. In the United States, it affects about 2,000 individuals annually and constitutes around 7% of liver transplants, while in the Far East, it accounts for more than two-thirds of liver transplants. Over the past decades, the causes of ALF have shifted, with a decline in hepatitis A and B cases and an increase in paracetamol overdose in Western countries. Drug-induced liver injury (DILI) is also a major cause in these regions, while viral infections like hepatitis E and B are more common in South Asia and parts of Hong Kong and Australia.

Prevention

Preventing ALF, particularly in Western countries, involves addressing the rising cases of paracetamol overdose. Efforts to curb access to over-the-counter paracetamol, along with clearer overdose warnings and alternative pain management options, are key preventive measures. Hepatitis A and B vaccination provides secondary prevention, though its effectiveness diminishes in patients with decompensated cirrhosis or post-liver transplantation.

Clinical Features

Taking a thorough patient history is crucial, focusing on potential exposures to viral infections or toxins. If the patient presents with severe encephalopathy, obtaining a collateral history may be necessary. Physical examination should assess mental status and look for signs of chronic liver disease (CLD). Jaundice is frequently observed but not always present. Right upper quadrant tenderness may also be present, though liver palpation can be difficult in cases of massive hepatocyte loss. Hepatomegaly may occur early in viral infections or conditions like congestive heart failure or Budd-Chiari syndrome. It is important to rule out signs of cirrhosis, as it has distinct management implications.

Differential Diagnosis

ALF can be caused by viral infections or drugs, with differences in incidence between regions. In the West, drug-induced ALF is more common, accounting for 19% to 75% of cases. In India, viral hepatitis causes 91% to 100% of ALF cases. Idiosyncratic drug reactions are particularly prevalent in developed countries, contributing to 13% of cases in the United States and 5% in the UK. Common drugs responsible for ALF include antibiotics, antivirals, antidepressants, anticonvulsants, immunosuppressants, and non-steroidal anti-inflammatory drugs (NSAIDs). DILI typically presents subacutely with lower aminotransferases and elevated bilirubin, with a poor prognosis and frequent need for liver transplantation. Infectious diseases, such as malaria, typhoid fever, leptospirosis, and dengue fever, can mimic ALF, especially in tropical regions or in travelers.

Clinical Investigations

Initial laboratory investigations focus on determining the etiology and severity of ALF. Tests include viral hepatitis serologies (HAV IgM, HBV surface antigen, HCV IgM), autoimmune markers (antinuclear antibodies, smooth muscle antibodies), and ceruloplasmin levels. Plasma ammonia, preferably arterial, can also provide insight. A liver biopsy may be needed for suspected conditions like autoimmune hepatitis, metastatic liver disease, or herpes simplex hepatitis. Additional tests, such as HIV status, are required in certain cases, especially when liver transplantation is considered.

Criteria for Diagnosis

ALF should be suspected in any patient with acute liver dysfunction and prolonged prothrombin time/international normalized ratio (INR) exceeding 1.5, accompanied by encephalopathy. The condition is defined by liver impairment and coagulation abnormalities (typically INR $\geq$ 1.5) with mental status changes in patients without prior cirrhosis, lasting less than 26 weeks. This includes patients with Wilson's disease, vertically acquired hepatitis B, or autoimmune hepatitis, provided their condition is diagnosed within this timeframe.

Treatment

The cornerstone of ALF management is intensive care, with a focus on identifying and treating the underlying cause. Prognosis heavily depends on this. Mortality in ALF is often due to sepsis, multiorgan failure, and intracranial hypertension. ALF typically involves circulatory disturbances characterized by vasodilation, which can cause renal failure and decreased systemic vascular resistance. Emergency liver transplantation is the only proven life-saving intervention. In addition to transplantation, intensive care support, fluid management, metabolic balance, infection prevention, and nutritional support are critical components of care. Regular monitoring of coagulation parameters, blood counts, metabolic panels, and liver function tests is essential, although changes in transaminases do not correlate directly with prognosis.

General Measures

Managing ALF requires vigilant monitoring for respiratory, haemodynamic, neurological, and gastrointestinal complications. Securing the airway with intubation may be necessary as patients lose the ability to protect it due to coma. Central venous access and blood pressure monitoring are crucial for assessing vascular status. Urinary catheterization is used to monitor renal function, and fluid resuscitation should be tailored to pulmonary pressures. Vasopressors like norepinephrine may be needed to maintain blood pressure. Managing hypoglycemia, hypokalemia, and other metabolic disturbances is vital in preventing further complications.

Likely Developments Over the Next 5 to 10 Years

1. N-acetylcysteine (NAC) in Non-Paracetamol Acute Liver Failure (ALF)

The role of N-acetylcysteine (NAC) is expected to expand beyond its traditional use in paracetamol-induced ALF. Evidence suggests that NAC could play a significant role in managing non-paracetamol-related ALF due to its antioxidant properties and potential to reduce liver damage. Further research will clarify its efficacy and the optimal dosing regimen.

2. Mild Hypothermia for Brain Oedema in ALF

Mild hypothermia is being explored as a therapeutic strategy to prevent or treat brain oedema in patients with ALF. Preliminary studies show that cooling the body could reduce intracranial pressure and improve outcomes, particularly in patients with elevated ammonia levels or severe hepatic encephalopathy. More rigorous clinical trials are needed to validate its benefits and establish safe protocols.

3. Optimal Biocomponents for Liver Support Devices

The development of liver support devices is focused on improving the biocomponents used in these systems. Identifying the optimal materials and components for artificial liver devices will be crucial for enhancing their ability to support liver function in patients with ALF. Future research will focus on optimizing these biocomponents to improve biocompatibility and efficiency.

4. Hepatocyte Progenitor Cells in Hepatocyte Transplantation

Hepatocyte progenitor cells, including fetal liver cells, multipotent hepatic cells, and bone marrow-derived stem cells, are being studied for their potential in liver transplantation. These cells may offer a viable alternative to full liver transplants by acting as functional hepatocytes. Research into these cells could provide new avenues for hepatocyte transplantation, offering less invasive options and better patient outcomes.

5. Auxiliary Partial Orthotopic Liver Transplantation (APOLT) as a Bridge

Auxiliary partial orthotopic liver transplantation (APOLT) is being investigated as a bridge to either full liver transplantation or spontaneous recovery in ALF patients. This technique involves transplanting only a portion of a donor liver, providing short-term support while the patient's liver may regenerate. This approach could be an effective interim solution, reducing the need for full transplants and improving patient survival.

6. Artificial and Bioartificial Liver Support Systems

Artificial and bioartificial liver support systems are evolving as potential lifesaving tools for patients with ALF. These devices, which include filtration and adsorption technologies, aim to remove accumulated toxins and support liver function. The future of these systems lies in their refinement to provide more efficient detoxification and better integration with the patient's physiological processes.

Controversies

1. Penicillin G and Silibinin for Mushroom Poisoning

The use of Penicillin G and silibinin (milk thistle) as antidotes for mushroom poisoning remains controversial. Although these agents have shown some promise in clinical trials, their effectiveness is still debated. Penicillin G is thought to inhibit the toxins in certain mushrooms, while silibinin may protect the liver. More robust studies are required to establish their clinical efficacy.

2. Selection of Patients for Liver Transplantation

The criteria for selecting patients for liver transplantation, particularly in cases of ALF, continue to be debated. There is no universal consensus on the best predictive models for outcomes, and the decision-making process can be highly individualized. Ongoing research will aim to refine selection criteria and ensure that transplants are offered to those most likely to benefit.

3. Bridging Options for Transplantation

The role and efficacy of bridging therapies for patients awaiting liver transplantation remain under scrutiny. Several options, including liver support devices and auxiliary partial liver transplants, are being explored to stabilize patients until a donor organ becomes available.

The challenge lies in determining which bridging therapies offer the best outcomes, and for which patients these interventions are most appropriate. More evidence is needed to guide clinical practice.

Chapter 14
Hematochezia and Lower Gastrointestinal Bleeding (LGIB)

Essentials

1. Hematochezia in Older Patients
Haematochezia, the passage of fresh blood in the stool, is frequently observed in individuals over 50 years of age. It can lead to hypovolemic shock if the blood loss is substantial.

2. Common Causes of Lower GI Bleeding by Age
In younger patients (under 50 years), anorectal conditions are the most prevalent cause of lower gastrointestinal bleeding. In contrast, diverticular disease is the leading cause in older adults.

3. Self-limiting Nature of Most Lower GI Bleeds
The majority of lower gastrointestinal bleeds are self-limiting, often resolving on their own without the need for intervention.

4. Initial Management in the Emergency Department

The primary focus in managing acute lower GI bleeding in the emergency department is on resuscitating the patient and evaluating potential risk factors for adverse outcomes.

5. Upper GI Bleeding Evaluation in Severe Cases

In cases of significant or massive bleeding, an esophagogastroduodenoscopy (OGD) is recommended to identify potential bleeding sources in the upper gastrointestinal tract.

6. Diagnostic Challenges

Despite advancements in diagnostic imaging, a bleeding source may remain unidentified in approximately 10% to 20% of cases.

Introduction

Hematochezia, defined as the passage of red blood or clots per rectum, is a hallmark symptom of lower gastrointestinal bleeding (LGIB), which occurs in the GI tract distal to the ligament of Treitz. This differs from upper gastrointestinal bleeding (UGIB), where blood typically presents as melaena, characterized by black, tarry stools due to oxidized hemoglobin.

The severity and presentation of hematochezia depend on the underlying cause and the speed of the bleeding, with episodes ranging from mild and intermittent to massive. Patients may also experience occult bleeding, leading to signs of anemia. The emergency management of hematochezia involves three key objectives:

1. Identifying the underlying cause and determining the bleeding's severity through a focused history, physical examination, and diagnostic tests.

2. Resuscitating and stabilizing the patient's hemodynamic status.

3. Coordinating with specialist teams for definitive diagnosis and treatment.

Aetiology

Several conditions can lead to hematochezia, with the incidence varying by age. Hemorrhoids are the leading cause in patients under 50 years. In a review of cases requiring hospitalization or colonoscopy for significant bleeding, diverticular disease was identified as the most common cause (17%–40%), followed by angiodysplasia (2%–30%), inflammatory or ischaemic colitis (9%–21%), and colonic neoplasia (11%–14%). In patients under 50, anorectal conditions like hemorrhoids and anal fissures contribute 4%–10% of cases. In up to 25% of patients, the source of bleeding remains unidentified.

Diverticulosis

Diverticulosis involves the formation of colonic diverticula, where mucosa and submucosa herniate through the bowel wall at weak points. The descending and sigmoid colon are most commonly affected, though right-sided diverticulosis is more frequent in Asian populations. Diverticulosis carries a bleeding risk of up to 48%, often due to the rupture of vasa recta. Risk factors include atherosclerosis, hypertension, smoking, steroid use, and NSAIDs. The typical presentation involves painless, acute hematochezia, which resolves spontaneously in 70%–80% of patients. However, 25%–30% of individuals may experience recurrent bleeding.

Angiodysplasia

Angiodysplasia is the abnormal dilation of blood vessels within the mucosal and submucosal layers of the GI tract, commonly in the proximal colon. It accounts for 2%–30% of LGIB cases, especially in patients over 65. Unlike diverticular bleeding, angiodysplasia often presents with self-limiting re-bleeding in 80% of untreated cases. Vascular anomalies, such as arteriovenous malformations, hemangiomas, and telangiectasias, are rarer and tend to occur in younger patients.

Enterocolitis

Enterocolitis refers to inflammation of the small bowel and colon, most often caused by infections. In these cases, fever, abdominal pain, tenesmus, vomiting, and diarrhea are predominant. Haematochezia may occur during diarrheal episodes, particularly with bacterial or parasitic infections, such as those caused by Escherichia coli, Shigella, Salmonella, Campylobacter , and Entamoeba . Severe forms of viral infections, like dengue or Ebola, can also cause hemorrhagic enterocolitis.

Ischaemic Colitis

Ischaemic colitis results from inadequate mesenteric blood flow, often affecting areas like the splenic flexure or rectosigmoid junction. It is more common in older patients with vascular risk factors such as atherosclerosis, hypertension, diabetes, and cardiac arrhythmias. Younger patients may develop ischaemic colitis due to vasculitis, drug use (e.g., cocaine), sickle cell anemia, or intense physical activity. The typical presentation includes acute abdominal pain followed by hematochezia within 24 hours. Radiation-induced enterocolitis is another potential cause, often following cancer treatments like prostate brachytherapy.

Inflammatory Bowel Disease (IBD)

In up to 50% of ulcerative colitis cases, patients may experience rectal bleeding, usually alongside prolonged diarrhea and loss of appetite. In contrast, Crohn's disease may cause less prominent hematochezia, although it can still lead to significant bleeding in some cases.

Neoplasia

Colorectal cancers are a common cause of occult or recurrent bleeding, especially in patients over 50. These neoplasms often present with additional symptoms like weight loss, abdominal pain, or changes in bowel habits. Post-polypectomy bleeding can also occur, typically within days to weeks following polyp removal.

Anorectal Disorders

Hemorrhoids are the most frequent cause of hematochezia, typically presenting as self-limiting episodes that respond to conservative treatment. Although rectal varices are rare, they can occur in patients with portal hypertension. Other anorectal conditions, including anal fissures, fistulas, abscesses, and trauma, may also result in bleeding. These are usually self-limiting and are treated by addressing the underlying condition.

Aortoenteric Fistula

Aortoenteric fistulas are rare complications of abdominal aortic aneurysm repair or untreated aneurysms eroding into the GI tract. These fistulas are typically located in the duodenum and present with a triad of abdominal pain, sepsis, and GI bleeding. A "herald bleed" may precede catastrophic hemorrhage.

Human Immunodeficiency Virus (HIV)

HIV infection rarely causes hematochezia but poses a diagnostic challenge due to its association with both common and HIV-specific GI conditions, such as cytomegalovirus-induced vasculitis, Cryptosporidium enteritis, and Kaposi's sarcoma of the GI tract.

Miscellaneous Causes

Medications, including NSAIDs and antiplatelet agents (e.g., aspirin and clopidogrel), can increase the risk of drug-induced hematochezia by exacerbating pre-existing conditions like diverticulosis. Anticoagulants like warfarin also complicate bleeding risks. Inherited or acquired bleeding disorders should be considered in the differential diagnosis.

Clinical Features

History

The patient's description of the bleeding is critical for determining its origin. Haematochezia is typically bright red and suggests lower GI tract bleeding, whereas bleeding from the right colon or jejunum may produce darker stools. However, stool color is not always reliable for distinguishing LGIB from UGIB, as transit time through the GI tract influences stool appearance. A history of haematemesis or "coffee ground" vomitus may suggest an upper GI source.

Vascular bleeding, such as from hemorrhoids or diverticula, is usually painless, whereas inflammatory or ischaemic causes are often associated with abdominal pain, tenesmus, diarrhea, or constipation. Colorectal cancer may cause painless bleeding, and a careful history may reveal other symptoms, such as weight loss and altered bowel habits. The acuity and volume of blood loss are often difficult for patients to estimate accurately.

Management of Hematochezia: Risk-Based Approach

The management of patients presenting with hematochezia (rectal bleeding) is guided by their risk profile, focusing on hemodynamic stabilization, identifying the bleeding source, and formulating an appropriate intervention plan (Fig. 7.13.1).

High-Risk Patients

For patients presenting with signs of significant blood loss or in hemorrhagic shock, immediate stabilization is critical. These patients should be placed under continuous cardiac and hemodynamic monitoring in the emergency department (ED). The initial approach involves ensuring airway, breathing, and circulation, with a focus on optimizing oxygen delivery. The first-line fluids for volume replacement are crystalloids or colloids, administered as an initial fluid challenge of 500 mL over 30 minutes. The volume of subsequent fluid resuscitation should be tailored based on the patient's response and clinical status.

For patients who do not respond to the initial fluid challenge, blood products are considered the preferred solution. In cases of massive blood transfusion, platelet and fresh frozen plasma administration should also be considered. Any coagulopathic state should be immediately addressed with interventions such as vitamin K, fresh frozen plasma, or prothrombin complex concentrates.

If the patient is on anticoagulant therapy, the decision to reverse anticoagulation should be weighed against the potential risk of thromboembolic events. This decision requires a multidisciplinary approach, with input from the relevant specialties involved in patient care. The primary goal is to normalize blood pressure and heart rate prior to proceeding with endoscopic interventions.

Moderate-Risk Patients

Patients with moderate or persistent non-massive bleeding should be admitted for close monitoring. They typically require colonoscopy within 24 hours. Preventive measures to reduce the risk of re-bleeding, such as avoiding NSAIDs or reassessing the need for anticoagulation reversal, should be considered during management.

Low-Risk Patients

Patients with mild, intermittent bleeding are often diagnosed with anorectal conditions. Those at higher risk for re-bleeding (e.g., patients over

60 years old with comorbidities, a history of diverticulosis or angiodysplasia, or recent hospitalization or colonoscopy for lower gastrointestinal bleeding) should be observed closely, with consultation for potential surgical intervention. Patients with lower-risk profiles may be discharged with appropriate follow-up care and referral to surgical or gastroenterology services. Colonoscopy is generally recommended for patients over 50 years old.

Definitive Investigations and Management

Colonoscopy Colonoscopy is the gold standard for diagnosing and managing lower gastrointestinal bleeding (LGIB). An urgent colonoscopy performed within 8 hours of presentation has a higher likelihood (74%-82%) of identifying the bleeding source compared to delayed procedures (48 hours), with the added benefit of enabling tissue diagnosis and therapeutic interventions, such as adrenaline injection, bipolar coagulation, or hemoclipping. Colonoscopy is particularly effective in managing active diverticular bleeding (70%-100% success rate) or post-polypectomy bleeding (95%-100% success rate). Adequate bowel preparation is essential for the procedure's success.

Esophagogastroduodenoscopy (OGD) In patients with severe hematochezia, approximately 11%-15% may have upper gastrointestinal (GI) tract lesions, making it worthwhile to consider OGD either prior to or simultaneously with colonoscopy, especially when no source is identified via colonoscopy.

Computed Tomography Angiography (CTA) CTA is useful for localizing the bleeding source in patients who are hemodynamically unstable or unable to undergo bowel preparation for colonoscopy. The sensitivity of CTA in detecting active bleeding is high (91%-92%) but drops to 45%-47% for intermittent bleeding.

Angiography Selective mesenteric angiography has traditionally been used to localize the bleeding source when colonoscopy is ineffective. During this procedure, contrast is injected into the superior mesenteric artery, inferior mesenteric artery, and coeliac trunk. A positive result is indicated by the extravasation of contrast. The sensitivity of angiography varies (27%-86%) and is more effective when the bleeding rate exceeds 0.5 mL/min. Embolization via a microcatheter can be performed to stop the bleeding with success rates of 80%-100%. If embolization is not possible, vasopressin infusion is considered as a second-line treatment.

Technetium-Labeled Red Blood Cell Scintigraphy There is ongoing debate regarding the usefulness of tagged red blood cell (99mTc RBC) scintigraphy in localizing GI bleeding prior to angiography. Although it may increase the diagnostic yield of angiography, its sensitivity for accurately identifying the bleeding source is moderate (65%-80%). Tagged RBC scintigraphy is particularly useful for intermittent or obscure overt GI bleeding and may guide angiography if positive.

Other Imaging Modalities

Magnetic Resonance Imaging (MRI): Primarily used for rectal cancer staging, providing detailed imaging of local prognostic factors.

Endoscopic Ultrasound (EUS): The modality of choice for evaluating small, superficial tumors.

Positron Emission Tomography (PET): While its role is not fully established, PET shows promise for detecting GI malignancies with high sensitivity and specificity.

Wireless Capsule Endoscopy (WCE): WCE is the preferred method for visualizing small bowel bleeding when previous diagnostic methods, including OGD and colonoscopy, fail.

Surgical Intervention

Surgical intervention for acute UGIB should be reserved for cases where all other therapeutic options have been exhausted. The decision should consider prior bleeding control measures, the severity of the bleeding, the source of the bleeding, and the patient's overall health status. Careful localization of the bleeding site is critical to avoid complications such as re-bleeding during surgery.

Controversies in Antiplatelet and Anticoagulant Therapy

The decision to continue or discontinue antiplatelet and anticoagulant medications following an episode of LGIB is complex and should involve a multidisciplinary team. For patients who have undergone coronary stenting, discontinuing clopidogrel within the first 30 days increases the risk of death and myocardial infarction. The risk associated with clopidogrel discontinuation remains high during the first 90 days following an acute coronary syndrome. However, for patients with more distant coronary interventions, discontinuing clopidogrel for up to 7 days while continuing aspirin therapy may be safe.

Chapter 15
Perianal Conditions Management

Essentials

1. Anorectal Symptoms: Pain, bleeding, and masses are common complaints associated with various anorectal conditions. A thorough patient history and comprehensive anorectal examination are crucial for accurate diagnosis.

2. Initial Management of Haemorrhoidal Disease and Fissures: For mild, uncomplicated haemorrhoidal disease and perianal fissures, increasing dietary fiber intake and addressing constipation are effective first-line treatments.

3. Management of Anorectal Abscesses: Anorectal abscesses require incision and drainage. While this procedure can be performed safely in the emergency department for some cases, abscesses located supralevator,

intersphincteric, or ischiorectal should undergo formal surgical exploration and drainage in the operating theater.

4. Abscess Drainage and Antibiotics: Incision and drainage of cutaneous abscesses in immunocompetent, afebrile adults generally does not result in bacteraemia, so routine antibiotic prophylaxis is typically unnecessary.

5. Management of Irreducible Haemorrhoids: Irreducible hemorrhoids require urgent reduction, often followed by surgical intervention.

Anorectal Abscesses and Fistulae

Overview

Anorectal abscesses and fistulae represent both the acute and chronic stages of the same underlying condition. Typically, the infection originates in an anal gland, usually due to the occlusion of the crypts. Anorectal abscesses are more prevalent in men than in women, with a peak incidence between the ages of 20 and 40. Contributing factors include inflammatory bowel disease, infections, trauma, surgery, malignancy, radiation, and immunosuppression. It is estimated that approximately 20% of individuals who experience anorectal abscess will later develop a fistula, with rates higher in patients suffering from Crohn's disease. Fistulous tracts can be complex and often involve the anal sphincters, making their treatment particularly challenging. The management of anorectal fistula is typically handled by colorectal surgeons.

Symptoms

The primary symptom of an anorectal abscess is perianal pain, accompanied by swelling and fever in some cases. On examination, a tender, red, fluctuating mass is usually found in the anorectal region. The abscess may be classified based on its location within four potential anorectal spaces.

Types of Abscesses

1. Perianal Abscess Perianal abscesses typically present as a painful lump around the anal verge, often lateral and posterior. They usually result from an infected anal gland, although they can occasionally indicate Crohn's disease. Examination often reveals a red, indurated area with possible fluctuation, which may be suitable for incision and drainage in the emergency department (ED).

2. Ischiorectal Abscess Ischiorectal abscesses are larger and may not display obvious skin changes due to the compressibility of ischiorectal fat. Patients often present with fever and general malaise. The induration is usually more lateral, and the abscess may not point until later, which can make the initial diagnosis resemble cellulitis of the buttock.

3. Intersphincteric Abscess These abscesses form between the internal and external sphincters within the anal canal. They are associated with severe pain and can lead to urinary symptoms. There may be no visible swelling, and the abscess typically points within the anal canal, often rupturing spontaneously.

4. Supralevator Abscess Located above the levator ani, supralevator abscesses are often secondary to intra-abdominal conditions, such as diverticular disease or Crohn’s disease. The patient may present with fever, pain on defecation, and changes in bowel habits, although external inspection may show no abnormality. A rectal exam will typically reveal a firm, tender mass.

Treatment

The cornerstone of treatment for anorectal abscesses is incision and drainage. Antibiotics alone are not effective. Small abscesses, particularly perianal ones, can often be drained in the ED with local anesthesia. Various incision techniques—radial, curvilinear, or cruciate—may be used, each with varying risks related to further fistula development and sphincter damage. Larger abscesses or more complicated cases require treatment under general anesthesia by a colorectal surgeon to minimize complications such as fistula formation and sphincter damage. If fistulas are suspected, their presence can be confirmed through surgery, where the fistulous tracts are delineated. In selected cases, managing the fistula during the initial abscess treatment may reduce recurrence without increasing incontinence.

After drainage, the wound should be kept open to allow for healing from the bottom up, and a formal drain may be placed. Probing should be avoided to prevent creating new fistulae. Postoperative care includes regular sitz baths, wound dressing changes, and follow-up reviews. Antibiotics are generally unnecessary unless the patient has underlying conditions like diabetes, immunosuppression, or a prosthetic device, in which case they may serve as an adjunct.

Pilonidal Disease

Overview

Pilonidal disease is a recurrent, acquired condition affecting young adults, with a higher incidence in men. The condition is not related to anorectal abscesses but involves the migration of loose hair into the natal cleft, leading to irritation and inflammation. This results in the formation of a pilonidal sinus or abscess. The clinical spectrum ranges from acute abscesses to chronic conditions with recurrent abscesses and extensive sinus tracts. Risk factors include hirsutism, obesity, sedentary lifestyle, and local irritation.

Symptoms

Patients with pilonidal disease typically report a painful lump in the sacrococcygeal area, with or without purulent discharge. Systemic symptoms are uncommon. Upon examination, swelling, pain, and discharge in the natal cleft are typically observed, along with midline draining pits or sinuses. Occasionally, hair may protrude from a pit.

Treatment

Initial treatment for an acute pilonidal abscess involves incision (preferably off-midline) at the site of abscess pointing, followed by drainage and evacuation of pus and hair. This can be performed under local or general anesthesia. For many patients, no further treatment is required, and healing may occur within 10 weeks. However, up to 63% of patients may require additional surgery for recurrent or failed treatments.

In cases of chronic or recurrent pilonidal disease, more complex surgical procedures—such as excision, marsupialization of sinuses, or the use of fibrin glue—are reserved for patients who fail simpler treatments. These procedures involve longer healing times and extended hospital stays. Laser hair removal may help prevent recurrence, though shaving is associated with higher recurrence rates.

Hemorrhoids

Overview

Hemorrhoidal cushions are normal anatomical structures that help maintain anal continence. Hemorrhoidal disease occurs when these structures become symptomatic, presenting as bleeding, prolapse, pain, thrombosis, or pruritus. Contributing factors include constipation, prolonged sitting, pregnancy, and other conditions that increase intra-abdominal pressure. Hemorrhoids are classified into internal and external types, with internal hemorrhoids being classified into four grades based on prolapse severity.

Clinical Features and Diagnosis

The most common symptom of hemorrhoidal disease is painless bright red bleeding during defecation, typically observed on toilet paper or stool. Other symptoms may include pruritus, a sensation of incomplete bowel evacuation, or a tender lump. Severe pain is rare but warrants investigation for alternate causes such as colorectal malignancy.

Anoscopy is used to diagnose internal hemorrhoids, and the differential diagnosis should include conditions such as colorectal cancer, inflammatory bowel disease, and anal warts. Patients with any suspicious findings, or those over 40 with a family history of cancer, should undergo further evaluation, including colonoscopy.

Treatment

Conservative treatments for hemorrhoidal disease focus on relieving constipation and reducing straining. Increasing dietary fiber intake has been shown to reduce symptoms significantly, particularly bleeding. Stool softeners, sitz baths, and topical treatments such as glyceryl trinitrate (GTN) paste can help alleviate symptoms by relaxing the anal sphincter and improving blood flow.

For specific cases such as prolapsed irreducible hemorrhoids or thrombosed external hemorrhoids, conservative measures may be insufficient. In these instances, surgical options, including excision or incision, may be considered. Thrombosed external hemorrhoids typically resolve with conservative measures, though excision may offer quicker relief if performed within 48 hours.

Procedural Treatment

Surgical treatments are indicated for more advanced hemorrhoidal disease, including grade 3 or 4 hemorrhoids or those that have failed conservative management. Options include rubber-band ligation, sclerotherapy, infrared photocoagulation, and more invasive procedures like hemorrhoidectomy or stapled hemorrhoidopexy. Although these procedures can be effective, they are associated with postoperative pain and bleeding.

Controversies in Anorectal and Perianal Management

Selection of Anorectal Abscesses for ED Drainage: When considering the drainage of anorectal abscesses in the emergency department (ED) under local anesthesia, how should we determine which cases are appropriate for this approach?

Management of Thrombosed External Hemorrhoids: Should thrombosed external hemorrhoids be treated with early excision, or is conservative management a more suitable option?

Long-Term Strategy for Pilonidal Disease: What is the most effective long-term treatment plan for managing pilonidal disease?

Effectiveness of Botulinum Toxin vs. Other Treatments for Acute Anal Fissures: Is botulinum toxin more effective than glyceryl trinitrate (GTN) ointment and topical calcium channel blockers in the treatment of acute anal fissures?

Role of Antibiotics in Perianal Suppurative Conditions: What, if any, is the role of antibiotics in the management of perianal suppurative diseases?

Selection Criteria for Foreign Body Removal in the ED: What factors should be considered when determining which foreign bodies are appropriate for attempted removal in the emergency department?

References

1. Abcarian, H. (2011). Anorectal infections: abscess-fistula. Clinical Colon and Rectal Surgery, 24(1), 14-21.

2. Sahnan, K., Askari, A., Adegbola, S.O., et al. (2017). The natural history of anorectal sepsis. British Journal of Surgery, 104(13), 1857-1865.

3. Rakinic, J. (2017). Anorectal abscess. BMJ Best Practice. Retrieved from http://bestpractice.bmj.com. Accessed January 31, 2018.

4. Ho, Y.H., Tan, M., Chui, C.H., et al. (1997). Randomized controlled trial of primary

fistulotomy with drainage alone for perianal abscesses. Diseases of the Colon & Rectum, 40(12), 1435-1438.

5. Rickard, M.J. (2005). Anal abscesses and fistulas. ANZ Journal of Surgery, 75, 64-72.

6. McCallum, I.J.D. (2017). Pilonidal disease. BMJ Best Practice. Retrieved from http://bestpractice.bmj.com. Accessed January 31, 2018.

7. Bendewald, F.P., Cima, R.R. (2007). Pilonidal disease. Clinical Colon and Rectal Surgery, 20(2), 86-95.

8. Aydede, H., Erhan, Y., Sakarya, A., Kumkumoglu, Y. (2001). Comparison of three methods in the surgical treatment of pilonidal disease. ANZ Journal of Surgery, 71(6), 362-364.

9. Thaha, M.A., Steele, R.J.C. (2017). Hemorrhoids. BMJ Best Practice. Retrieved

from http://bestpractice.bmj.com. Accessed January 31, 2018.

10. Alonso-Coello, P., Guyatt, G., Heels-Ansdell, D., et al. (2005). Laxatives for the treatment of hemorrhoids. Cochrane Database of Systematic Reviews, 4, CD004649.

11. Tjandra, J.J., Tan, J.J., Lim, J.F., et al. (2007). Rectogesic (glyceryl trinitrate 0.2%) ointment relieves symptoms of hemorrhoids associated with high resting anal canal pressures. Colorectal Disease, 9(5), 457-463.

12. Altomare, D.F., Rinaldi, M., La Torre, F., et al. (2006). Red hot chili pepper and hemorrhoids: the explosion of a myth—results of a prospective, randomized, placebo-controlled, crossover trial. Diseases of the Colon & Rectum, 49(7), 1018-1023.

13. Chan, K.K., Arthur, J.D. (2013). External hemorrhoidal thrombosis: evidence for current

management. Techniques in Coloproctology, 17(1), 21-25.

14. Lohsiriwat, V. (2015). Treatment of hemorrhoids: a coloproctologist's view. World Journal of Gastroenterology, 21(31), 9245-9252.

15. Nelson, R.L., Thomas, K., Morgan, J., Jones, A. (2012). Non-surgical therapy for anal fissure. Cochrane Database of Systematic Reviews, 2, CD003431.

16. Gandomkar, H., Zeinoddini, A., Heidari, R., Amoli, H.A. (2015). Partial lateral internal sphincterotomy versus combined botulinum toxin A injection and topical diltiazem in the treatment of chronic anal fissure: a randomized clinical trial. Diseases of the Colon & Rectum, 58(2), 228-234.

17. Nelson, R.L., Chattopadhyay, A., Brooks, W., et al. (2011). Operative procedures for fissure in . Cochrane Database of Systematic Reviews, 11, CD002199.

18. Heard, S. (2004). Pruritus ani. Australian Family Physician, 33(7), 511-513.

19. Atkin, G.K., Suliman, A., Vaizey, C.J. (2011). Patient characteristics and treatment outcomes in functional anorectal pain. Diseases of the Colon & Rectum, 54(7), 870-875.

20. Ayantunde, A.A. (2013). Approach to the diagnosis and management of retained rectal foreign bodies: clinical update. Techniques in Coloproctology, 17(1), 13-20.

21. Ostrowski, K., Edwards, G., Maruno, K. (2016). Removal of retained rectal foreign bodies in the emergency department. Emergency Medicine Australasia, 28(4), 459-465.

www.ingramcontent.com/pod-product-compliance
Lightning Source LLC
Chambersburg PA
CBHW071449220526
45472CB00003B/736

9798300629267